D1326729

The Slimming Foodie

IN ONE

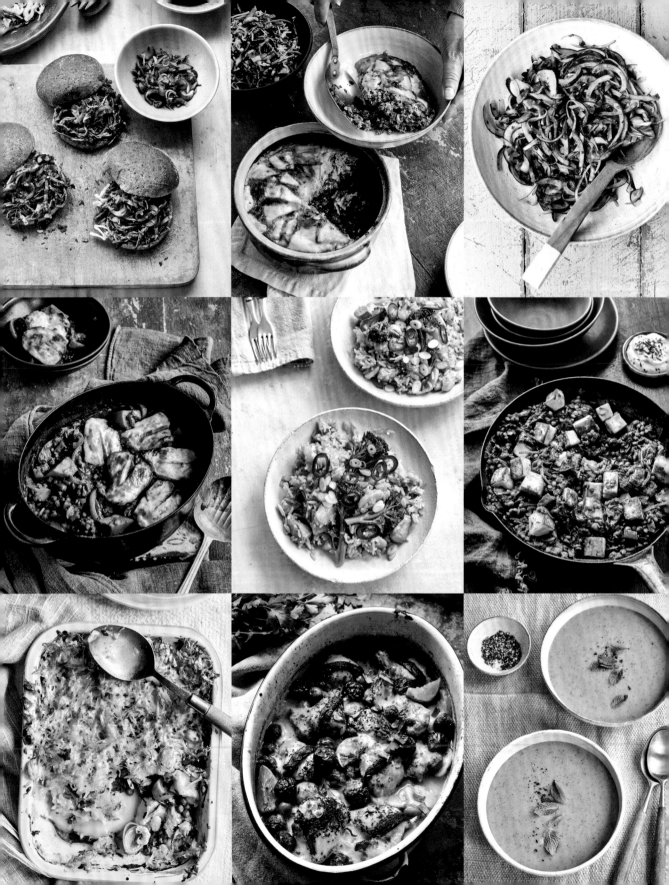

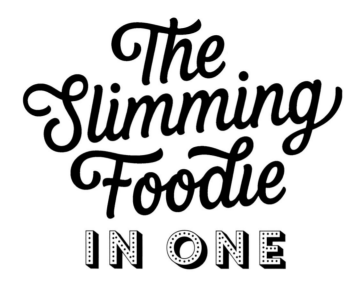

The Slimming Foodie

IN ONE

PIP PAYNE

100+ ONE-DISH RECIPES UNDER 600 CALORIES

ASTER*

First published in Great Britain in 2022 by Aster,
an imprint of Octopus Publishing Group Ltd
Carmelite House
50 Victoria Embankment
London EC4Y 0DZ
www.octopusbooks.co.uk

An Hachette UK Company
www.hachette.co.uk

Text copyright © Pip Payne 2022
Photography copyright © Chris Terry 2022
Design and layout copyright © Octopus Publishing
Group 2022

All rights reserved. No part of this work may be reproduced
or utilized in any form or by any means, electronic or
mechanical, including photocopying, recording or by
any information storage and retrieval system, without
the prior written permission of the publisher.

Pip Payne asserts her moral right to be identified as the
author of this work.

ISBN 978 1 78325 499 6

A CIP catalogue record for this book is available from the
British Library.

Printed and bound in China
10 9 8 7 6 5 4 3 2 1

Senior Commissioning Editor: Natalie Bradley
Senior Managing Editor: Sybella Stephens
Copy Editor: Lucy Bannell
Art Director: Yasia Williams-Leedham
Designer: www.gradedesign.com
Photographer: Chris Terry
Food Stylists: Henrietta Clancy, Georgie Besterman,
  Octavia Squire
Props Stylist: Tamsin Weston
Senior Production Manager: Katherine Hockley

Author's notes:
The information contained in this book is not intended
to replace any dietary advice from your own qualified
nutritionist or dietician. Any application of the ideas and
information contained in this book is at the reader's sole
discretion and risk.

Both imperial and metric measurements have been given
in all recipes. Use one set of measurements only and not
a mixture of both.

 Suitable for vegetarians

 Freezer friendly

CONTENTS

INTRODUCTION

The most popular dishes on my blog, The Slimming Foodie, are always one-pot recipes. This makes complete sense, as most of us cook in a hurry day-to-day and not only do we not want to faff around with multiple pans, but we don't want to wash them up either!

I think that a true one-pot dish uses a single vessel to cook the whole meal. You might need some bowls for preparation, or to use a food processor, but you aren't cooking with any more than one pan, or pot, or tray, or slow-cooker. I regard it as a bit of cheat when something is labelled 'one-pot' but then you have to cook rice or potatoes separately. I always strive to make my recipes as straightforward and fuss-free as possible.

All of the meals in this book are designed to be able to be eaten on their own without extra cooked side dishes. That doesn't mean, however, that you can't cook extra sides with them. Lots of the meals would work well over rice, or would be complemented by green vegetables, a side salad or some bread if you prefer them that way or want the meal to go further.

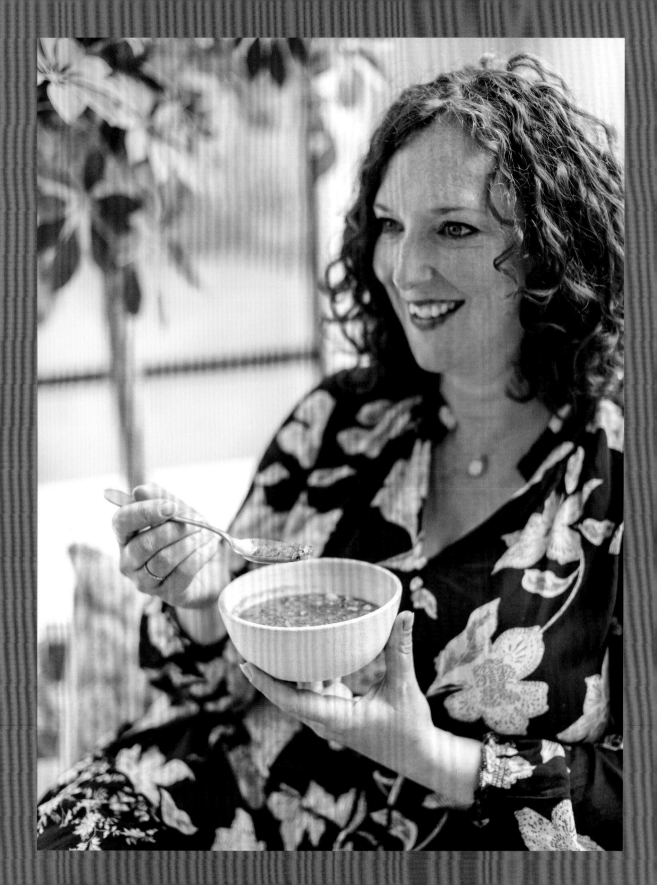

I have organized this book into seven chapters to reflect
my methods of one-dish cooking:

IN A POT

Cooked in a pot or pan, on the hob and in the oven,
or in the oven only.

IN A PAN

Cooked in one pan on the hob only.

IN A TRAY

Traybaked, oven dish and roasting tin meals
all cooked in the oven.

SOUP-ER

Soups for any mood.

IN A SLOW-COOKER

Some slow-cooker winners.

ALL IN THE PREP

Easy salads, side dishes and (mostly) recipes that
don't need cooking.

JAZZ IT UP

My top homemade condiments/spice mixes/sauces…
anything that jazzes up home cooking!

I have included a good balance of vegetarian, meat and fish dishes, as well as a variety of pasta, grain, potato, bean and vegetable recipes. Some of the meals are more indulgent than others, but all of them come in at less than 600 calories per serving. My recipes are nearly always easily adaptable to accommodate you and your family's tastes and preferences; I suggest throughout how to tweak meat dishes to be vegetarian (and vice versa), point out easy vegetable swaps or additions, and make serving suggestions.

You might be using this book without watching the calories, in which case please feel free to use full-fat versions of yogurt, coconut milk and crème fraîche, or use extra cheese, butter or oil – these certainly won't ruin any of the recipes, but obviously may take them above 600 calories.

I hope that you can find cooking inspiration and new family favourites in this book, as well as easy ways to cook from scratch and save time in the kitchen. I love to see all the versions of my recipes cooked by my online community, so please feel free to join in on all my social media platforms and share what you are cooking.

WHAT KITCHEN EQUIPMENT DO I NEED?

POTS, PANS & DISHES

I have used just a few different dishes for all the meals in the book, and here are the essentials:

- **A casserole dish with a lid:** I have a nonstick dish which is so helpful for meals where you need to fry ingredients first. I have small (20cm/8 inch), medium (24cm/9½ inch) and large (26cm/10½ inch) versions, but just one medium dish will be fine.
- **Roasting tins:** I use cheap stainless-steel tins for most of my oven baking, which are versatile and easy to clean. I have small (26 × 20cm/10½ × 8 inch), medium (34 × 24cm/13½ × 9½ inch) and large (40 × 32cm/16 × 12½ inch) versions.
- **Ovenproof dish:** I use this for meals such as oven-baked risotto or couscous. The one I use most is an ovenproof glass rectangular dish/roaster (which has a super-handy lid for storing the food afterwards), measuring 24 × 19cm (9½ × 7½ inch).
- **Sauté pan:** One of my most-used saucepans, essentially a deep frying pan with a lid.
- **Loaf tin** (900g/2lb)
- **Nonstick square cake tin** (23cm/9 inch)
- **12-hole muffin tin**

APPLIANCES

For convenience, I rely on a few staple kitchen appliances which make home-cooking so much easier and more time-efficient.

- **Slow-cooker:** These can be great value and they are so handy. I use a 3.5-litre (6¼-pint) slow-cooker.
- **Mini chopper:** There are a few recipes in this book which require this, which looks like a mini food processor and is incredibly useful for curry pastes and sauces. These are inexpensive and make such a difference to the preparation of food, saving you from lots of fine chopping or having to use a pestle and mortar.
- **Food processor:** I find this so useful for making sauces or dips and for grating or shredding.
- **Blender:** For years I have had a cheap supermarket own-brand blender, which I use regularly for making soups.

BITS & BOBS

- **A good-quality sharp knife:** One of the most important things. A blunt knife makes preparing vegetables and meat such a chore. It's really worth investing in a decent knife, as, if you are cooking, you will use it every day.

- **Measuring spoons:** Important for accuracy and for adhering to the calorie counts.

- **Kitchen scales:** For confidence in portions of ingredients such as rice and pasta, these are invaluable.

- **Large and small mixing bowls:** A range of sizes will help you in a variety of tasks, from making dough to mixing salad dressings.

- **Microplane:** I much prefer to use this for zesting than a regular zester, as it's more efficient, and zests fruit more finely. It's also really handy for Parmesan cheese.

HELPFUL TIP

Look out for these symbols at the top of each recipe page:

 SUITABLE FOR VEGETARIANS

 FREEZER FRIENDLY

GENERAL COOKING NOTES

- **Oil:** I usually specify spray oil because that's what I mainly cook with. I have a refillable spray bottle that I fill with olive oil. I also use low-calorie cooking spray, particularly for things I'm baking in the oven, as it can give such good coverage in just a few sprays. If you prefer to use only cooking spray, then that will work for all the recipes in this book.

- **Calories:** The calorie counts stated in the recipes are for a single portion and do not include serving suggestions or side dishes. Calorie calculations can vary based on the precision of your measurements, the brand of ingredients or the source of nutrition data. The information provided is intended as only a guide.

- **Pans and dishes used:** I sometimes suggest a specific size of pan or dish, and if you use a different size, cooking times may vary. In recipes where I do not specify a particular size, it is because it is less important and it shouldn't affect the overall dish if you use a different size.

- **Portion sizes:** Obviously, these vary hugely form person to person and family to family. I have based my portion sizes both on recommended portions and personal experience of cooking for my family. You may need to adjust these to work for your own family. I have also suggested side dishes for meals, if you're feeling hungry.

- **Freezing:** My suggestions for freezer-friendly meals are based on my preferences. When freezing meals, always allow the food to fully cool before placing in the freezer. I usually transfer leftovers into airtight plastic containers or freezer bags, then label them with the contents and date. Food should be thoroughly defrosted before reheating. Leaving food to defrost in the refrigerator overnight will allow it to defrost at a safe temperature.

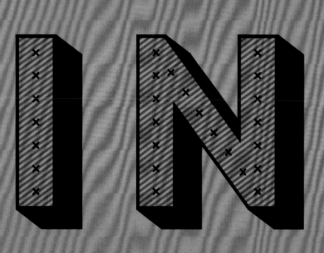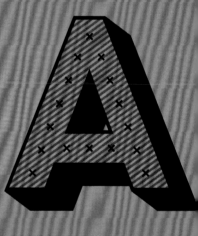

CHAPTER 1

IN A

POT

TUSCAN BUTTER BEAN BAKE

Bursting with Italian flavour, with a hearty and filling vegetarian base of butter beans. You can serve this up with a simple rocket salad with balsamic vinegar.

CALORIES PER SERVING: 320
PREP TIME: 10 MINUTES
COOK TIME: 30 MINUTES

spray oil
1 red onion, finely chopped
1 red pepper, deseeded and finely
    chopped
2 garlic cloves, crushed
250g (9oz) chestnut
    mushrooms, quartered
200g (7oz) cherry tomatoes
1 teaspoon fennel seeds
2 teaspoons smoked paprika
2 tablespoons Italian herb mix
2 × 400g (14oz) cans of butter
    beans, drained and rinsed
150ml (¼ pint) water
3 tablespoons tomato purée
1 tablespoon balsamic vinegar
100g (3½oz) kale, finely sliced
30g (1oz) Parmesan-style
    vegetarian cheese, grated
150g (5½oz) mozzarella cheese,
    torn
salt and pepper
handful of parsley leaves,
    to serve

1. Preheat the oven to 220°C/200°C fan (425°F), Gas Mark 7.
2. Spray a medium-large flameproof casserole dish with oil and fry the onion and pepper for 5 minutes.
3. Add the garlic, mushrooms, cherry tomatoes and fennel seeds and stir-fry for 5 more minutes. Spoon in the smoked paprika and Italian herb mix, then season with salt and pepper. Tip in the butter beans, measured water, tomato purée and balsamic vinegar, then stir in the kale and bring up to a simmer.
4. Stir through the Parmesan-style vegetarian cheese, then remove the dish from the heat, scatter the mozzarella over the top and place on the top shelf of the oven for 15 minutes, until the cheese is melted and bubbling.
5. Grind some pepper over the bake and scatter on some fresh parsley before serving.

NOTE To spice it up, add a finely chopped red chilli with the garlic in step 3. For a non-vegetarian version, fry some Italian sausage or chunks of pork fillet with the onion and pepper in step 2.

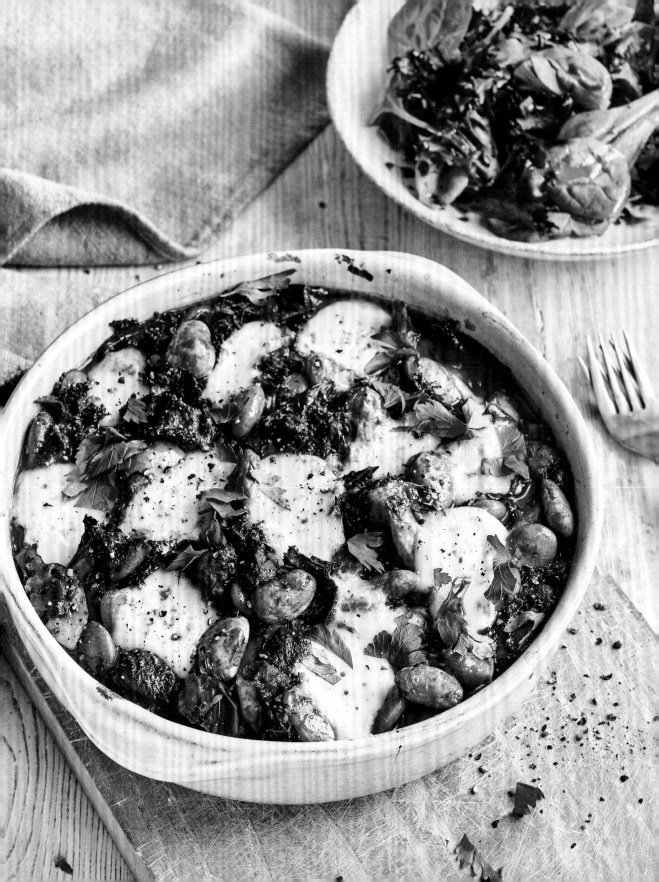

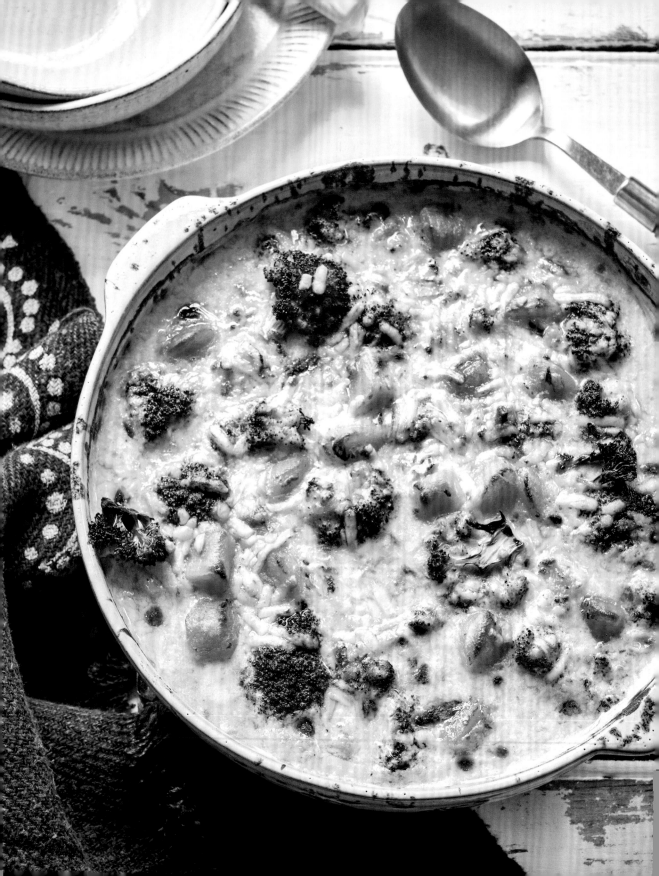

BUBBLING GNOCCHI BROCCOLI CHEESE

Gnocchi, little Italian dumplings, are a great ingredient to pick up for a quick, tasty dinner. I think they work so well in cheesy bakes, and this one is really irresistible. A savoury, creamy cheese sauce bubbles away with gnocchi, haricot beans and broccoli for a dish that tastes far more indulgent than it really is!

CALORIES PER SERVING: 472
PREP TIME: 10 MINUTES
COOK TIME: 30 MINUTES

500ml (18fl oz) semi-skimmed milk
500g (1lb 2oz) fresh gnocchi
400g (14oz) can of haricot beans, drained and rinsed
100g (3½oz) light cream cheese
250ml (9fl oz) vegetable stock
½ teaspoon onion granules
½ teaspoon garlic granules
florets from a head of broccoli, broken into bite-sized pieces
120g (4¼oz) mature Cheddar cheese, grated
salt and pepper

1. Preheat the oven to 220°C/200°C fan (425°F), Gas Mark 7.
2. Pour the milk into a deep flameproof casserole dish and bring it up to a simmer.
3. Add the gnocchi and haricot beans and simmer for 2 minutes. Stir in the cream cheese and simmer for a further 5 minutes, stirring constantly.
4. Add the stock, onion granules, garlic granules, broccoli and about half the Cheddar and stir it all together. Season with salt and pepper. Bring to the boil, then remove from the heat and sprinkle the remaining cheese over the top.
5. Pop the pot into the oven, near the top, and bake for 20 minutes, or until the cheese on top is browning and bubbling.

NOTE You can turn this into a gorgeous cheesy tuna bake. Simply add a can of drained tuna in spring water at the same time as the broccoli in step 4 and stir it in thoroughly. You can also spice the recipe up with 1 teaspoon of chilli flakes. If you want to increase the amount of vegetables, try adding cauliflower florets to the sauce for a cauliflower cheese vibe.

SWEET POTATO & LENTIL CURRY
WITH HALLOUMI

This recipe is inspired by a jalfrezi, which classically contains a meat, such as chicken, along with peppers, onions, tomatoes and spices. To make this vegetarian version I have added cubes of sweet potato and green lentils for a hearty and filling meal. Sizzling, salty halloumi grilled on top adds great texture and flavour.

CALORIES PER SERVING: 394
PREP TIME: 15 MINUTES
COOK TIME: 65 MINUTES

spray oil
1 onion, finely chopped
3 garlic cloves, crushed
2 red chillies, deseeded and finely chopped
3 sweet peppers (red, orange or yellow), deseeded and sliced
400g (14oz) can of chopped tomatoes
3 tablespoons tomato purée
300ml (½ pint) hot vegetable stock
400g (14oz) can of green lentils, drained and rinsed
1 sweet potato, peeled and chopped
210g (7½oz) halloumi cheese, sliced
1 teaspoon chilli flakes, to serve

FOR THE SPICE MIX
2 teaspoons ground cumin
2 teaspoons garam masala
2 teaspoons ground turmeric
1 teaspoon ground ginger
1 teaspoon salt

1. Prepare the spice mix by mixing all the ingredients together in a small bowl.
2. Spray a large flameproof and ovenproof dish (with a lid) with oil and fry the onion for 8 minutes until translucent and softly golden.
3. Add the garlic, chillies and peppers and fry for 5 minutes. Add the spice mix and stir-fry for 1 minute to coat all the vegetables. Add the chopped tomatoes, tomato purée, hot stock, lentils and sweet potato. Give everything a thorough stir, place the lid on the pot and leave to simmer gently for 40 minutes.
4. Stir the curry. If it is looking very liquid, increase the heat to high and bubble it hard for a couple of minutes to evaporate some of the liquid.
5. Preheat a grill to its highest setting.
6. Remove the pot from the heat and place the halloumi over the top. Place the pot under the hot grill for 8–10 minutes until the halloumi is brown and bubbling but not burned. Sprinkle over some chilli flakes before serving.

NOTE This is a great way to use up leftover roast meat, just slice it up and add it in step 3 after the curry has been bubbling away for 30 minutes. If you'd like to add fresh meat to this, you could use chicken breast, lamb leg steaks or frying beef. Add the meat in step 3, then follow the recipe.

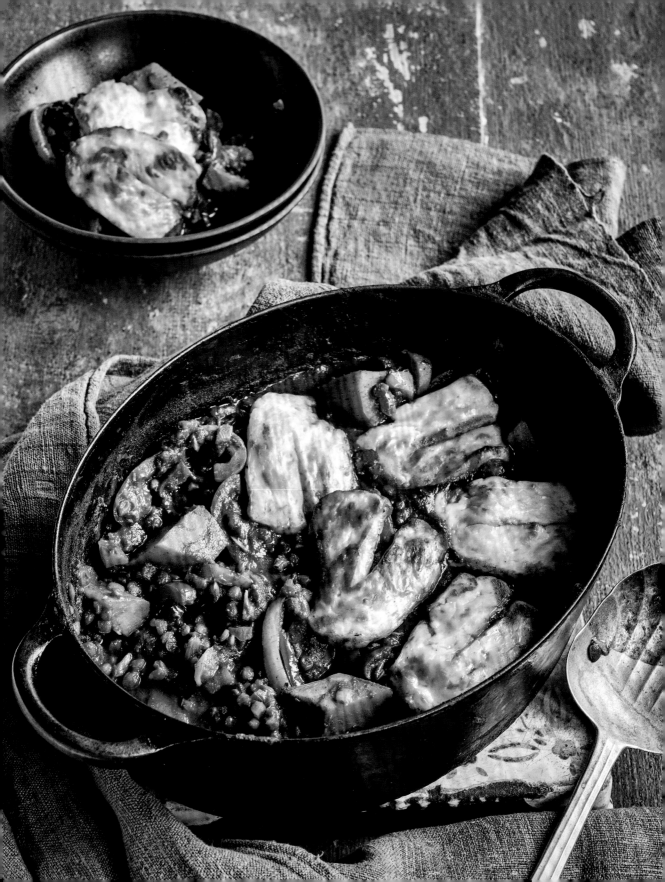

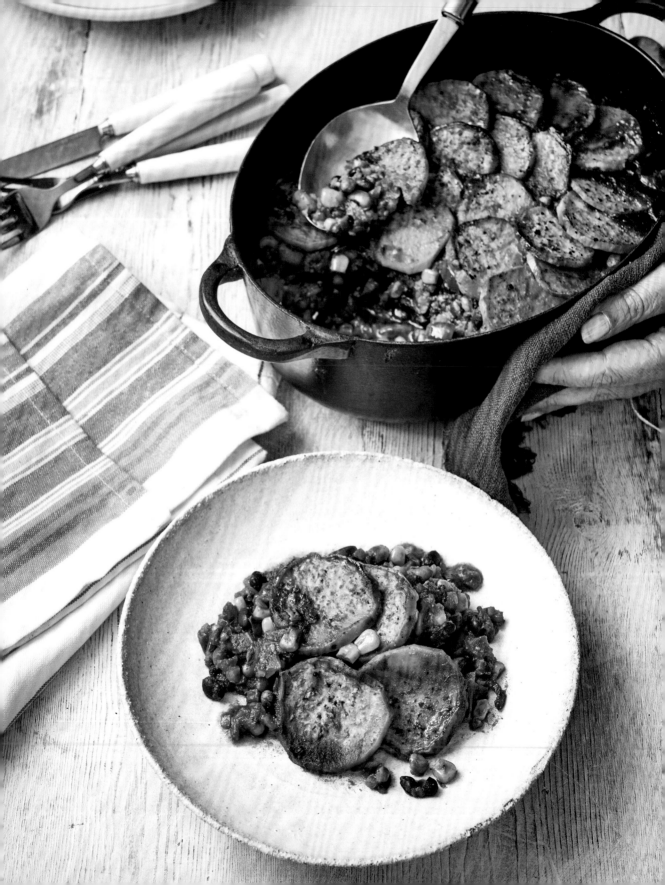

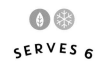

CHILLI BEAN PIE

Here, Mexican-inspired beans and vegetables are baked under sliced sweet potatoes to form a hotpot-style dish. Serve with sliced avocado, crunchy shredded lettuce and lime juice, or Quick Purple Pickle (see page 210).

CALORIES PER SERVING: 238
PREP TIME: 15 MINUTES
COOK TIME: 45 MINUTES

spray oil
2 red onions, finely chopped
2 celery sticks, finely chopped
3 garlic cloves, crushed
2 red peppers, deseeded and finely
    chopped
400g (14oz) can of chopped tomatoes
400g (14oz) can of black beans,
    drained and rinsed
400g (14oz) can of pinto beans,
    drained and rinsed
2 tablespoons tomato purée
150g (5½oz) frozen sweetcorn
1 tablespoon pickled jalapeños,
    finely chopped (optional)
200ml (7fl oz) boiling water
about 300g (10½oz) sweet
    potatoes, peeled and sliced into
    fine circles
paprika (any type), for sprinkling

FOR THE SPICE MIX
½ teaspoon chilli powder
1 teaspoon ground cumin
1 teaspoon dried oregano
1 teaspoon garlic granules
1 teaspoon sweet paprika
1 teaspoon salt
½ teaspoon pepper

1. Prepare the spice mix by mixing all the ingredients together in a small bowl. Preheat the oven to 220°C/200°C fan (425°F), Gas Mark 7.

2. Spray a flameproof casserole dish (mine was 24cm/9½ inches in diameter) with oil and fry the red onions for 8 minutes until soft. Add the celery, garlic and peppers and stir-fry for 5 minutes, then stir in the spice mix.

3. Add the chopped tomatoes, black beans and pinto beans, tomato purée, sweetcorn, jalapeños (if using) and measured boiling water, bring up to a simmer, then stir thoroughly.

4. Remove from the heat and lay the sweet potato slices over the top, starting in the middle and overlapping them in a circle until you reach the edge of the dish. Spray the top with spray oil or low-calorie cooking spray and sprinkle with a little bit of paprika.

5. Pop on to the middle shelf of the oven and bake for 30 minutes until the sweet potatoes are cooked through and golden brown.

NOTE You can customize the beans you use to fit in with your household's tastes – my favourites are black beans and pinto beans, but you could use more traditional kidney beans, or branch out to borlotti, butter beans or cannellini. This dish is easy to adjust for meat lovers, simply fry some chicken thigh fillets or lean minced beef after frying the onions in step 2 for a meatier chilli bean pie.

PIZZA MAC 'N' CHEESE

All the flavours of your favourite pizza in a very simple pasta recipe. Cook the macaroni in a tasty pizza sauce, then either mix in the pizza toppings, or add them on top with the bubbling cheese. This is a great way to accommodate fussy eaters, as you only add what they like. You can substitute another pasta shape, though please note that if you use a larger size than macaroni, you might need to add extra liquid as the pasta is cooking.

CALORIES PER SERVING: 508, WITHOUT TOPPINGS
PREP TIME: 5 MINUTES
COOK TIME: 30 MINUTES

500ml (18fl oz) tomato passata
250ml (9fl oz) semi-skimmed milk
150ml (¼ pint) water
1 teaspoon onion granules
1 teaspoon garlic granules
300g (10½oz) macaroni
1 teaspoon dried oregano
90g (3¼oz) Cheddar cheese, grated
100g (3½oz) mozzarella cheese, torn
toppings/fillings of choice (see note)
salt and pepper

1. Preheat the oven to 200°C/180°C fan (400°F), Gas Mark 6.
2. Pour the passata, milk and measured water into a small flameproof casserole dish (about 24cm/9½ inches in diameter), add both the onion and garlic granules and bring to the boil.
3. Add the macaroni, reduce the heat a little and allow to bubble away for 15 minutes, stirring occasionally to make sure the pasta does not clump together or stick to the bottom of the pot.
4. After 15 minutes, season to taste, add the oregano, then stir through half of each of the grated Cheddar and torn mozzarella.
5. Cover the top of the pasta with all the remaining cheese and pop into the oven for 15 minutes, until the cheese on top is bubbling and the macaroni is cooked through (if not, cook for 5 more minutes before checking again).

NOTE I haven't included extra 'toppings' to the main recipe, as it's a very personal choice! You could top the dish with anchovies (as I have done in the photo), jalapeños or bacon when it goes into the oven to melt the cheese, or stir in mushrooms, peppers, olives, pepperoni, sweetcorn or tuna with the cheese in step 4. If your favourite pizza topping is ham and pineapple, you could add those! (Please note that this dish is no longer vegetarian if you add pepperoni, tuna, anchovies or bacon, and that your toppings will increase the calorie count.)

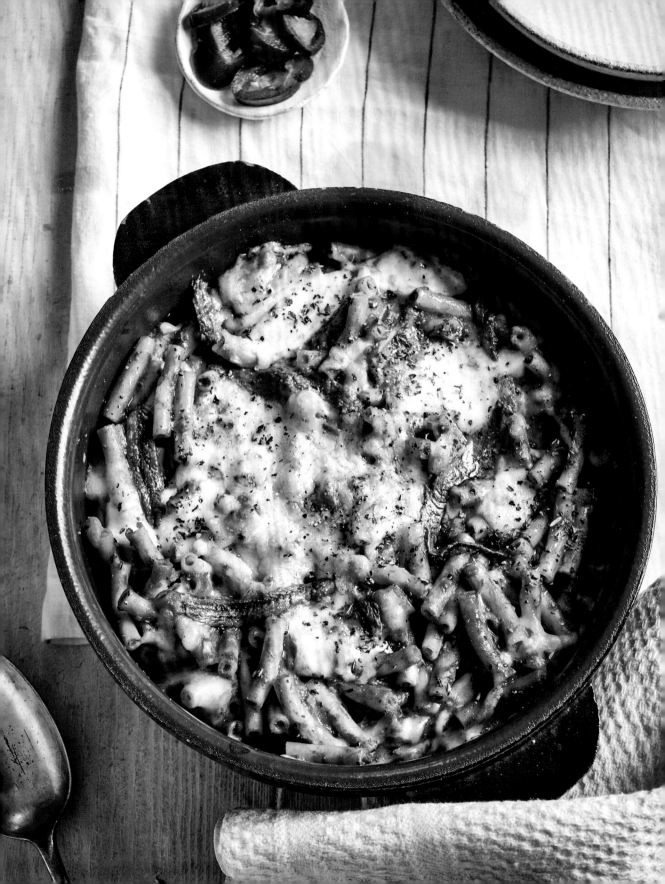

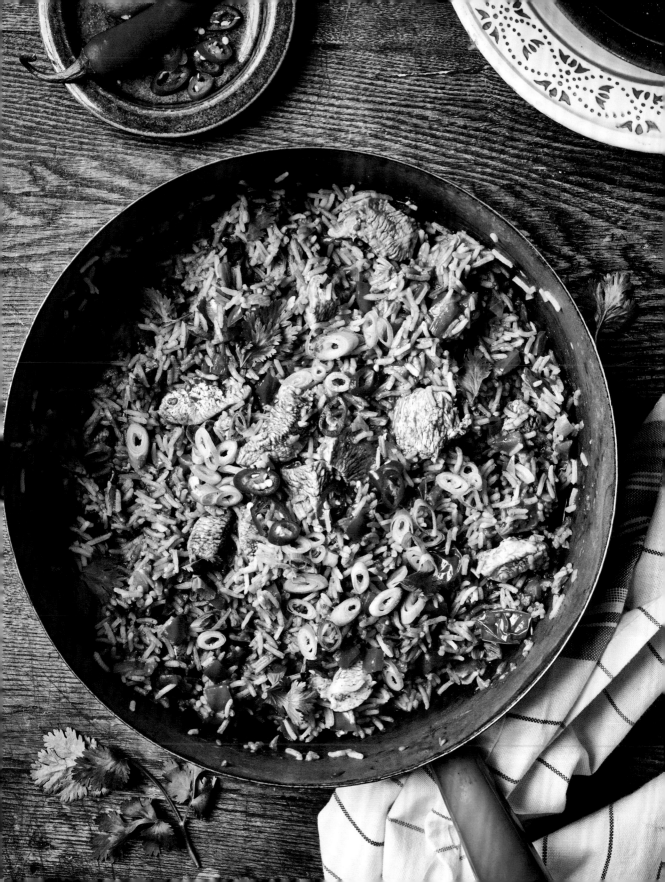

SAVOURY CHILLI CHOCOLATE RICE

One of my favourite Mexican dishes is chicken mole, which has a thick and delicious chilli-chocolate sauce. This one-pot rice recipe has the amazing flavours of a mole sauce, but it's much lighter, as well as a meal in one.

CALORIES PER SERVING: 423
PREP TIME: 15 MINUTES
COOK TIME: 30 MINUTES

spray oil
1 onion, finely chopped
2 garlic cloves, crushed
150g (5½oz) cherry tomatoes, halved
2 red peppers, deseeded and finely chopped
2 skinless chicken breasts, chopped small
250g (9oz) long grain white rice
600ml (20fl oz) hot chicken stock

FOR THE MOLE PASTE

1 tablespoon cocoa powder
1 tablespoon smooth peanut butter
1 tablespoon tomato purée
1 teaspoon honey
1 teaspoon chilli powder
½ teaspoon ground cinnamon
½ teaspoon ground cumin
½ teaspoon salt
½ teaspoon smoked paprika
juice of 1 lime

TO SERVE

coriander leaves
spring onions, finely chopped
red chilli, finely chopped
lime wedges

1. Preheat the oven to 200°C/180°C (400°F), Gas Mark 6.
2. Make the paste by mixing together all the ingredients in a small bowl until well combined.
3. Spray a large flameproof casserole dish (with a lid) with oil and fry the onion for 3 minutes, then add the garlic, tomatoes and peppers. Stir-fry for 5 minutes.
4. Add the chicken and the mole paste, then increase the heat and stir-fry for about 1 minute, giving the paste a chance to sizzle.
5. Stir in the rice, then the hot stock, stir again and place the lid on the pot. Put on to the middle shelf of the oven for 20 minutes to cook. Check the rice is ready (if not, allow it to simmer for longer, adding a little water if necessary). Remove from the oven and leave to rest for 5 minutes.
6. Stir thoroughly, then garnish with coriander, spring onions and red chilli and serve with lime wedges.

CHICKEN MOLE-STYLE SAUCE WITHOUT RICE

To make up a chicken mole-style sauce without adding the rice, follow steps 2–4, then add a 400g (14oz) can of chopped tomatoes and 150ml (¼ pint) water and allow to simmer for 25 minutes. You can then serve this over rice, or cauliflower rice.

MARK'S CHICKEN

Our friends Mark and Lorraine are true foodies and have been so helpful in sharing ideas for this book. Mark has kindly let me share his brilliant one-pot chicken dish. It's a taste of the Mediterranean with the flavours of garlic, lemon, anchovies and olives. Mark's original version contains chorizo, which I have swapped for tomatoes, but feel free to add it back as it is delicious!

CALORIES PER SERVING: 473
PREP TIME: 10 MINUTES
COOK TIME: 1¼ HOURS

500g (1lb 2oz) new potatoes, sliced lengthways (cut each potato into about 4, depending on size)

100ml (3½fl oz) hot chicken stock

8 chicken thigh fillets, fat trimmed away

8 anchovy fillets (from a can), drained and patted with kitchen paper to remove excess oil

16 pitted green olives in brine (from a jar)

2 lemons, each cut into 4 wedges lengthways

2 garlic cloves, finely sliced lengthways

150g (5½oz) cherry tomatoes, halved

½ teaspoon dried oregano

spray oil

100g (3½oz) mozzarella cheese, torn into small pieces

salt and pepper

1. Preheat the oven to 200°C/180°C fan (400°F), Gas Mark 6.
2. In a medium casserole dish (with a lid), layer the sliced new potatoes and pour over the chicken stock. Lay the chicken thighs over the potatoes in a circle and place an anchovy fillet on each thigh.
3. Scatter the olives over and place the lemon wedges around the chicken. Space the garlic slices evenly around the top of the dish, add the cherry tomatoes and sprinkle the oregano over everything. Season with salt and pepper, spray the top with spray oil, place the lid on the pan and bake in the oven for 1 hour.
4. Remove from the oven, scatter the mozzarella over the top, then return to the oven for 15 minutes until the mozzarella is golden and bubbling.
5. Serve straight away (don't eat the lemon pieces) and spoon over the pan gravy with each serving.

> **WHAT TO DO WITH LEFTOVER ANCHOVIES?**
> Make a delicious simple puttanesca pasta sauce!
> Fry 3 crushed garlic cloves, the remaining anchovy fillets and a finely chopped red chilli for 2–3 minutes until the anchovies have dissolved. Pour in a 400g (14oz) can of chopped tomatoes, add some halved and pitted olives (I usually use black but if you have green then those are good, too), season with salt and pepper and simmer for 25 minutes before mixing into hot al dente spaghetti.

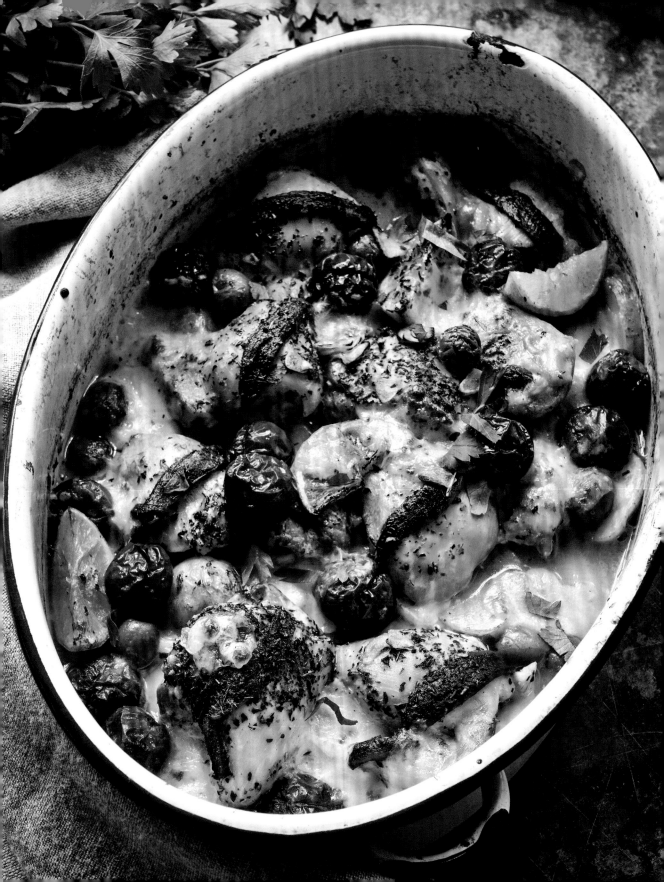

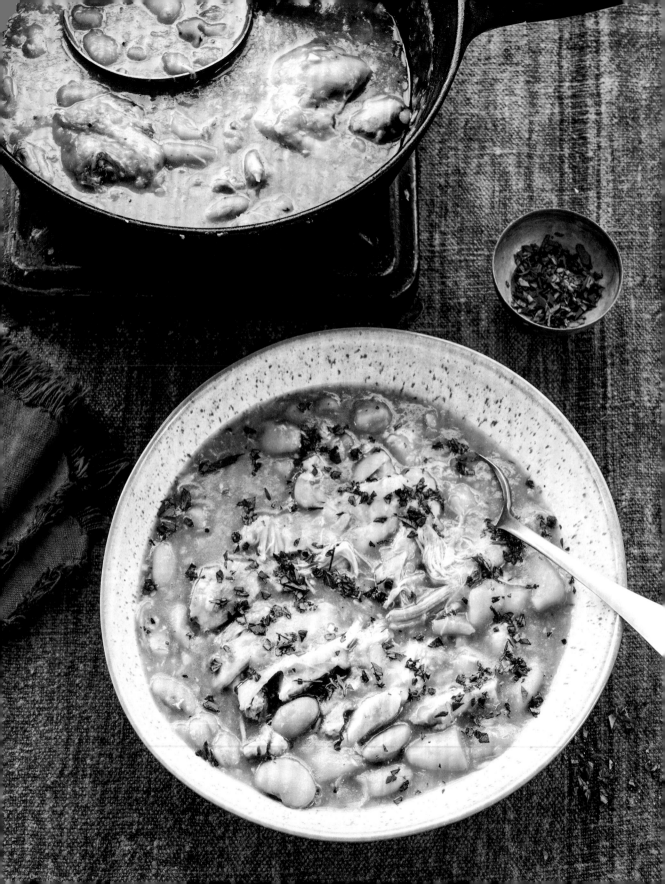

CHICKEN LEMON PEPPERPOT

I was inspired to make my own 'lemon pepper' after spending time with some great friends at a restaurant of that name in Spain and have found that it's a simple and versatile mix to have on hand. The deep warmth that the pepper adds to this dish is both satisfying and comforting, while a combination of fibre- and protein-rich butter beans and soft potatoes make for a filling meal.

If you are feeding this to children who may find the peppery taste too much, make the dish without adding the lemon pepper (just add some finely grated unwaxed lemon zest instead) and sprinkle the lemon pepper on as an optional seasoning when serving up.

CALORIES PER SERVING: 433
PREP TIME: 10 MINUTES
COOK TIME: 45 MINUTES

spray oil
6 chicken thigh fillets (about
   600g/1lb 5oz), fat trimmed
   away
1 large onion, finely chopped
4 garlic cloves, crushed
1½ tablespoons Lemon Pepper
   (see page 225)
1 tablespoon cornflour
1 litre (1¾ pints) hot chicken
   stock
450g (1lb) potatoes, peeled and
   cut into bite-sized chunks
400g (14oz) can of butter beans,
   drained and rinsed
juice of 1 lemon
small handful of parsley leaves,
   finely chopped

1. Spray a large, deep flameproof casserole dish (with a lid) with oil and fry the chicken thigh fillets over a medium heat for 5 minutes, until very little pink is showing on the outside.
2. Add the onion and garlic and fry for a further 5 minutes, stirring regularly.
3. Stir in the lemon pepper and cornflour.
4. Pour in the hot stock and add the potatoes and butter beans, place the lid on and simmer over a gentle heat for 30 minutes.
5. At the end of the cooking time, stir in the lemon juice, then remove the chicken thigh fillets and slice finely with a sharp knife before stirring back into the sauce. The sauce will thicken up as the chicken absorbs the liquid but if you wish to reduce the liquid, simply increase the heat and allow it to bubble and evaporate. Scatter with the parsley before serving.

NOTE If you'd like to increase the vegetables in the sauce, or use an alternative to the potato, parsnips or sweet potatoes work well in this dish.

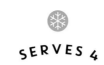

CHEAT'S COQ AU VIN BLANC

Smoked bacon, chicken and white wine form the base flavours of this delicious French-inspired casserole. Classic coq au vin is cooked in at least a whole bottle of wine (and usually red wine); this recipe still has that amazing flavour, but with much less wine. I've added new potatoes to make it an all-in-one meal, but if you can manage to add a bit of French bread to mop up the sauce, then all the better.

CALORIES PER SERVING: 458
PREP TIME: 15 MINUTES
COOK TIME: 1 HOUR 25 MINUTES

spray oil
1 onion, finely chopped
2 leeks, trimmed and sliced
3 smoked bacon medallions,
    finely chopped
3 garlic cloves, crushed
200g (7oz) button mushrooms
6 chicken thigh fillets
1 tablespoon cornflour
150ml (¼ pint) white wine
750ml (1 pint 7fl oz) hot chicken
    stock
1 teaspoon Dijon mustard
½ teaspoon dried thyme
2 carrots, peeled and sliced
500g (1lb 2oz) baby new potatoes
salt and pepper
chopped fresh parsley leaves,
    to serve

1. Spray a large, flameproof casserole (with a lid) with oil and stir-fry the onion, leeks, bacon, garlic, mushrooms and chicken for 10 minutes.

2. Add the cornflour and some salt and pepper and stir together with the ingredients in the pan. Pour in the wine and the hot stock, then mix in the mustard, thyme, carrots and potatoes.

3. Stir everything together thoroughly, then place the lid on the casserole and cook on the middle shelf of the oven for 1¼ hours.

4. Remove the casserole from the oven, stir thoroughly and shred the tender chicken a bit so it disperses through the casserole.

5. Serve with a grind of pepper and some fresh parsley.

NOTE Coq au vin goes really well with green veg such as asparagus, green beans or broccoli. To keep it all in one pot, simply add the vegetables at the end of the oven cooking time, pop the lid back on and simmer the pan on the hob for 5 minutes.

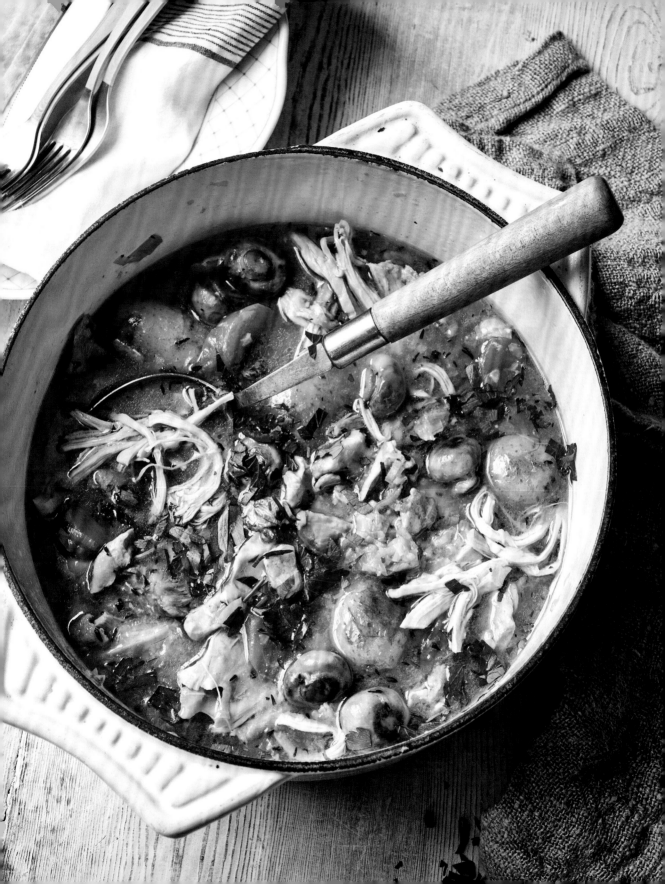

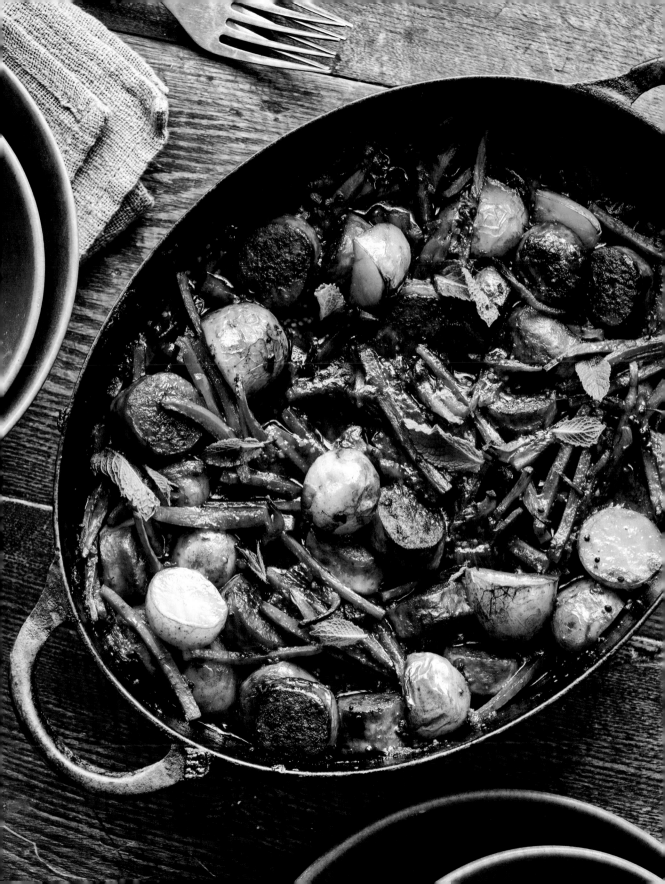

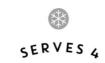

HONEY & MINT SAUSAGE HOTPOT

One of my favourite glazes for sausages is honey and mint. Here, I have brought those flavours into an all-in-one hotpot. The combination of honey, mint and mustard makes a sweet-and-savoury gravy for sausages, potatoes and carrots, which is irresistible and family friendly.

CALORIES PER SERVING: 308
PREP TIME: 15 MINUTES
COOK TIME: 50 MINUTES

spray oil
1 red onion, finely chopped
8 reduced-fat pork sausages,
    each cut into 6
2 garlic cloves, crushed
large handful of mint leaves
    (about 20g /¾oz), finely
    chopped, plus extra to serve
2 tablespoons red wine vinegar
2 tablespoons honey
1 tablespoon light soy sauce
1 litre (1¾ pints) hot beef stock
2 teaspoons wholegrain mustard
3 tablespoons tomato purée
450g (1lb) baby potatoes, halved,
    or quartered if large
300g (10½oz) carrots, peeled
    and cut into matchsticks
salt and pepper

1. Preheat the oven to 220°C/200°C fan (425°F), Gas Mark 7.
2. Spray a flameproof casserole dish with oil and fry the onion and sausage pieces over a high heat for 5 minutes, constantly stirring (don't worry if the sausages break a bit, this will help thicken the gravy).
3. Add the garlic, mint, vinegar, honey and soy sauce to the pan and stir-fry for 2 minutes, coating the sausage and onion and reducing the liquid slightly. Pour in the hot stock, stir, then add the mustard and tomato purée and mix to create the gravy.
4. Add the potatoes and carrots, season with salt and pepper, bring to the boil, then transfer to the middle shelf of the oven (uncovered) and cook for 40 minutes.
5. Give everything in the pot a thorough stir, then serve with mint scattered over the top.

NOTE This is a lovely easy dish to sneak in some more of the family's favourite vegetables! You could replace the potatoes with butternut squash or sweet potato, or add mushrooms. You could also thicken the sauce and bulk up the meal by adding dried red lentils at the same time as the stock.

WITH VEGGIE SAUSAGES
If you wish to use vegetarian sausages, then fry the onion on its own in step 2, then add the sausage pieces in step 3 with the garlic.

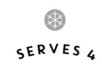

PIP'S IRISH LAMB & BARLEY STEW

Good, hearty, rustic comfort food. This stew has the filling power of both potatoes and barley, with lots of vegetables and a herby sauce. I use lamb leg steaks here because they are naturally quite lean and it is easy to trim away excess fat. I also use a fairly small amount of meat, both to keep it cost-effective and because the meal is as much about the vegetables and grain as the meat. If you want to increase the amount of meat, you can easily do so.

CALORIES PER SERVING: 378
PREP TIME: 20 MINUTES
COOK TIME: 1 HOUR 40 MINUTES

spray oil
300g (10½oz) lamb leg steaks, fat trimmed away , chopped quite small
1 onion, finely chopped
2 leeks, trimmed and sliced
2 celery sticks, finely sliced
2 garlic cloves, crushed
1.5 litres (2½ pints) hot beef stock
100g (3½oz) pearl barley
2 carrots, peeled and sliced
2 potatoes (total weight about 300g/10½oz), peeled and cut into bite-sized chunks
2 tablespoons tomato purée
1 teaspoon Dijon mustard
1 teaspoon dried rosemary
1 teaspoon dried thyme
salt and pepper
parsley leaves, to serve

1. Preheat the oven to 180°C/160°C fan (350°F), Gas Mark 4.
2. Spray a large flameproof casserole pot (with a lid) with oil. Fry the lamb for 2 minutes, then add the onion, leeks, celery and garlic. Fry over a medium heat for 8 minutes, stirring occasionally.
3. Add the hot stock, barley, carrots, potatoes, tomato purée, mustard, rosemary and thyme and season with salt and pepper. Stir everything together well.
4. Put the lid on the pan and place on to the middle shelf of the oven for 1½ hours. The sauce should be thick and rich and the lamb pieces tender. Serve scattered with parsley.

NOTE Try adding other vegetables, such as swede, turnip, butternut squash and sweet potato. You can also finely slice up cabbage to add to the sauce halfway through the cooking time. Or use lean diced beef as an alternative to lamb, if you prefer. Or even replace 500ml (18fl oz) of the stock with the same amount of stout, for a tasty little twist on the sauce, but bear in mind this will increase the calorie count..

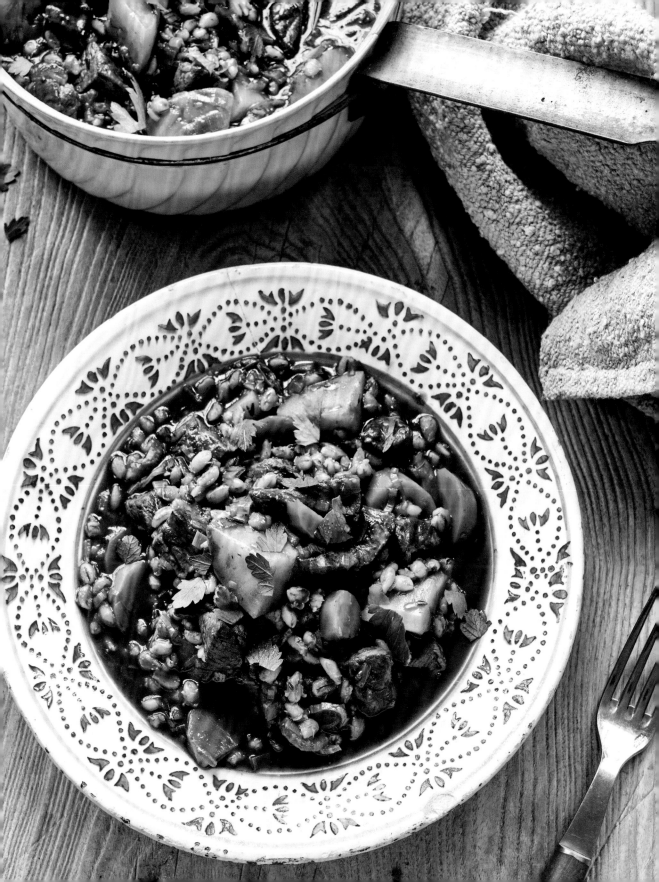

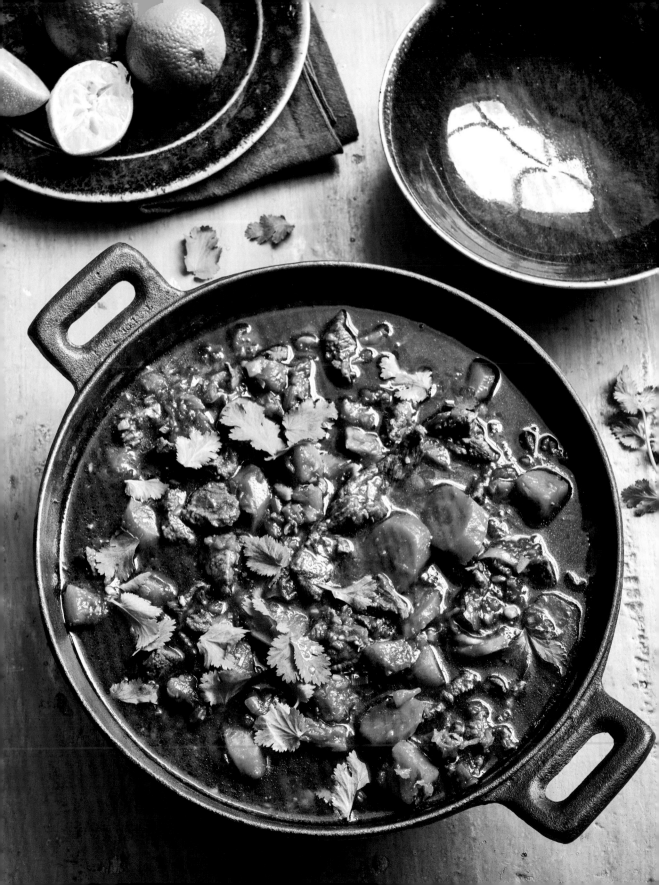

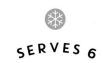
FRAGRANT BEEF & BUTTERNUT SQUASH STEW

A one-pot beef stew inspired by Vietnamese flavours. Butternut squash adds filling power and negates the need for a side dish, although this is also lovely served with rice if you want to make it go further.

CALORIES PER SERVING: 292
PREP TIME: 20 MINUTES
COOK TIME: 1 HOUR 40 MINUTES

spray oil
800g (1lb 12oz) lean beef, chopped
   into chunks
2 onions, finely chopped
2 garlic cloves, crushed
1 lemon grass stalk, trimmed and
   finely chopped (see page 150)
30g (1oz) fresh root ginger,
   peeled and grated
1 litre (1¾ pints) hot beef stock
1 tablespoon Chinese 5 spice
3 tablespoons tomato purée
2 tablespoons dark soy sauce
1 tablespoon fish sauce
3 carrots, peeled and sliced
1 butternut squash (about 1kg/
   2lb 4oz), peeled and chopped
   (see page 162), or 850g (1lb 14oz)
   prepared butternut squash

TO SERVE
coriander leaves
lime wedges

1. Preheat the oven to 180°C/160°C fan (350°F), Gas Mark 4.
2. Spray a large flameproof casserole dish (with a lid) with oil and stir-fry the beef and onions for 5 minutes. Add the garlic, lemon grass and ginger and stir-fry for 3 minutes.
3. Pour in the hot stock and add the Chinese 5 spice, tomato purée, soy sauce and fish sauce.
4. Stir in the carrots and butternut squash, place a lid on and put on the middle shelf of the oven. Cook for 1½ hours until the beef is tender.
5. Serve scattered with coriander, and with lime wedges on the side.

KEEPING GINGER FRESH
If you have a large piece of fresh root ginger and don't want to let any go to waste, simply pop it into a ziplock bag or airtight container and keep it in the freezer. It is easy to peel and grate when it is frozen, lasts much longer and will always be there when you need it.

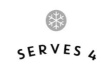

JUMBLED COTTAGE PIE

Cottage pie is an easy family favourite, but this version has layered potato slices instead of mashed potato, which allows the whole thing to be cooked as one. I grate in carrots and parsnip, which adds a sweet flavour to the sauce. This dish works really well with my Roast Brussels Sprouts with Balsamic & Honey (see page 191).

CALORIES PER SERVING: 598
PREP TIME: 15 MINUTES
COOK TIME: 1 HOUR 10 MINUTES

spray oil
1 onion, finely chopped
500g (1lb 2oz) extra-lean minced
    beef (less than 5 per cent fat)
2 carrots, peeled and grated
1 parsnip, peeled and grated
1 beef stock cube
4 tablespoons tomato purée
2 tablespoons Worcestershire
    sauce
1 tablespoon brown sauce,
    such as HP
1 teaspoon dried thyme
400g (14oz) can of baked beans
750g (1lb 10oz) potatoes, peeled
    and finely sliced
100g (3½oz) mature Cheddar
    cheese, grated
salt and pepper

1. Preheat the oven to 210°C/190°C fan (410°F), Gas Mark 6½.
2. Spray a large flameproof casserole dish (with a lid) with oil and fry the onion and minced beef for 5 minutes, breaking apart any lumps in the meat (I use a wooden spoon for this).
3. Add the grated carrots and parsnip, crumble in the stock cube and add the tomato purée, 1 tablespoon of the Worcestershire sauce, the brown sauce, thyme and baked beans. Season with salt and pepper and increase the heat until everything is bubbling. Remove the pan from the heat, then remove half the meat mixture into a bowl.
4. Smooth over what remains in the casserole dish with a large spoon, then layer in half the sliced potatoes to completely cover the mixture. Sprinkle on half the cheese. Now add the remaining meat mixture to cover the potatoes and cheese, again smoothing over the top. Layer the remaining potatoes neatly over the top, cover with the remaining grated cheese, then splash the remaining 1 tablespoon of Worcestershire sauce over the cheese.
5. Cover the pan and bake on the middle shelf of the oven for 45 minutes. Remove the lid and bake for a further 15 minutes. Serve immediately.

NOTE For added fibre, try halving the amount of beef and replacing it with a 400g (14oz) can of green lentils, drained and rinsed, adding them at step 3 with the baked beans. You can also use sliced sweet potato to replace the regular potato in this recipe, for an added twist.

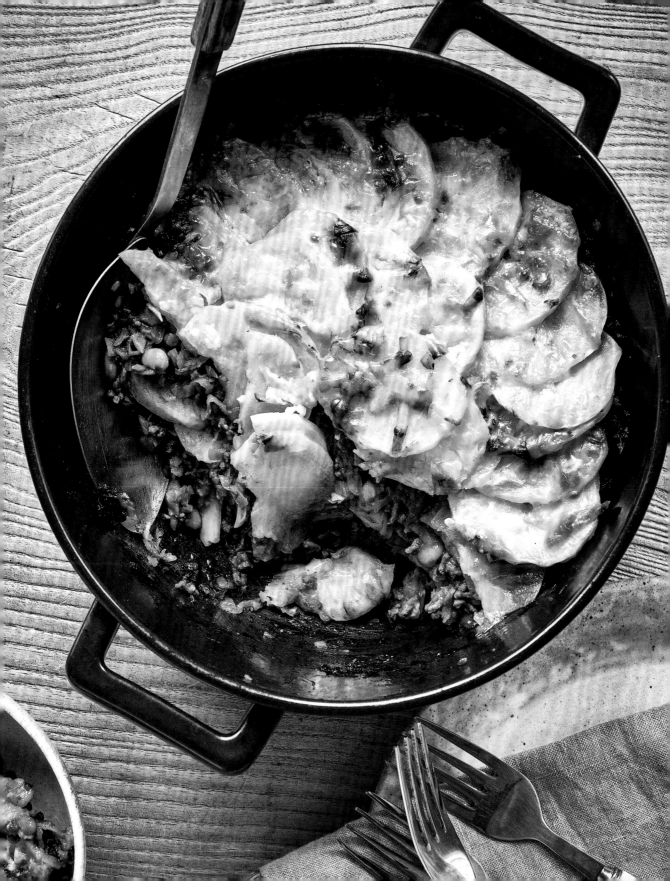

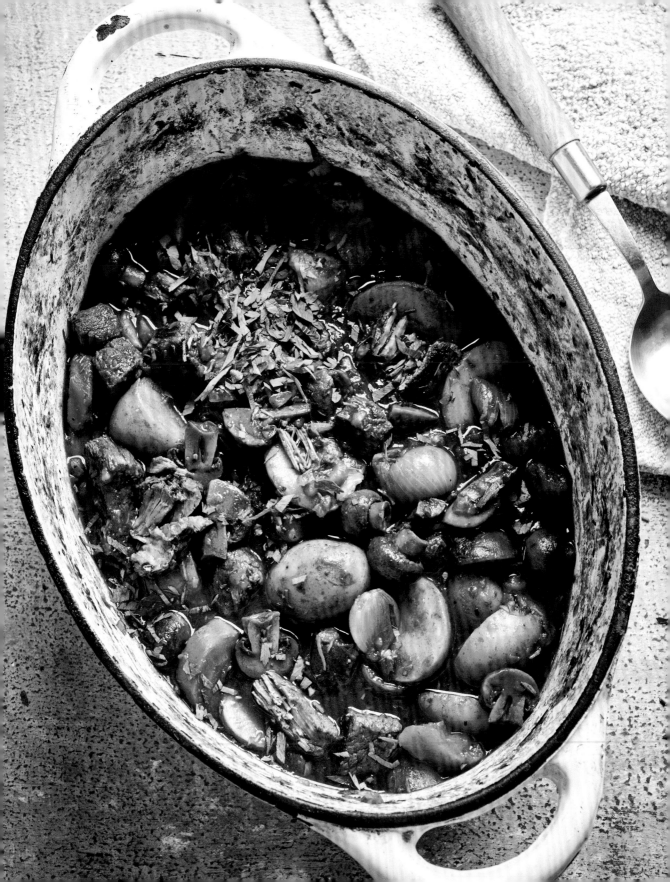

BEEF BOURGUIGNON

Beef Bourguignon has always been one of my top meals, but many traditional recipes use an entire bottle of red wine, as well as lots of oil, butter and bacon fat. My leaner version of the classic still has incredible, satisfying flavour, and I have also made it a meal-in-one by adding new potatoes, so there's no need for any additional side dishes. Although, when I cook this for friends and family, I usually add a lovely crusty loaf of French bread!

CALORIES PER SERVING: 512
PREP TIME: 20 MINUTES
COOK TIME: 2 HOURS 10 MINUTES

spray oil
3 celery sticks, finely chopped
3 bacon medallions (fat removed), finely chopped
12 shallots, peeled
600g (1lb 5oz) lean diced beef
4 garlic cloves, crushed
2 tablespoons cornflour
150ml (¼ pint) red wine
600ml (20fl oz) hot beef stock
3 tablespoons tomato purée
1 teaspoon dried thyme
1 teaspoon dried rosemary
1 teaspoon salt
1 teaspoon pepper
2 tablespoons dark soy sauce
4 carrots (total weight about 350g/12oz), peeled and sliced
250g (9oz) chestnut mushrooms, halved or quartered if large
650g (1lb 7oz) baby potatoes, larger ones halved so all are roughly the same size
parsley leaves, chopped, to serve

1. Preheat the oven to 200°C/180°C fan (400°F), Gas Mark 6.
2. Spray a large flameproof casserole dish (with a lid) with oil and stir-fry the celery, bacon and shallots over a medium heat for 3 minutes. Add the beef and garlic and stir-fry for a further 5 minutes to sear the outside of the beef.
3. Stir the cornflour through, then add the wine, hot stock, tomato purée, thyme, rosemary, salt and pepper, soy sauce, carrots and mushrooms to the pan. Gently mix everything together and bring up to a simmer. Place the lid on the pan and put on to the middle shelf of the oven for 1 hour.
4. After 1 hour, give everything a stir, add the baby potatoes to the pan, replace the lid and cook for 1 more hour.
5. Serve scattered with chopped parsley.

NOTE If you like, you can add swede or parsnip to this in step 4 at the same time as the potatoes to add filling power. You could also substitute those new potatoes for sweet potatoes or butternut squash, if you prefer.

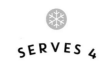

PHILLY CHEESESTEAK BAKE

The combination of flavours in a Philly cheesesteak is just spot on and, although delicious served the traditional way in a long bread roll, they also make a great stand-alone dish. The eggs work to hold the bake together, so it's easy to serve up. A hearty but low-carb recipe and a good way to use up any green peppers that are sitting around. This is great served with a big mixed salad, or my Super Slaw (see page 183).

CALORIES PER SERVING: 453
PREP TIME: 10 MINUTES
COOK TIME: 50 MINUTES

spray oil
2 onions, finely chopped
4 large eggs
50ml (1¾fl oz) semi-skimmed milk
1 tablespoon Worcestershire sauce
500g (1lb 2oz) lean minced beef (less than 5 per cent fat)
2 green peppers, deseeded and finely chopped
4 large flat mushrooms, roughly chopped
1 teaspoon onion granules
1 teaspoon garlic granules
½ teaspoon English mustard powder
1 beef stock cube
140g (5oz) Edam cheese, finely sliced
salt and pepper

1. Preheat oven to 200°C/180°C fan (400°F), Gas Mark 6.
2. Spray a small flameproof casserole dish or ovenproof frying pan (mine is about 20cm/8 inches in diameter) with oil and fry the onions for 10 minutes over a gentle heat until soft and golden brown.
3. Meanwhile, beat the eggs in a medium-sized bowl with the milk, Worcestershire sauce and some salt and pepper.
4. Increase the heat under the casserole dish, add the beef, peppers and mushrooms and stir-fry with a wooden spoon, breaking up the clumps in the meat while you brown it, for about 5 minutes. Add the onion granules, garlic granules and mustard powder and crumble over the stock cube. Stir well and remove the pan from the heat.
5. Pour the egg mixture over, making sure you cover all the exposed beef mix, then lay the slices of cheese on top.
6. Put the casserole dish on to the middle shelf of the oven and bake for around 35 minutes, until the cheese on top is bubbling and golden brown. Serve up while piping hot.

NOTE Fancy a bit of spice in this? Mix 1 tablespoon of chilli sauce with the egg mixture in step 3 before pouring it over the meat. If you have leftovers, try serving them up in a bread roll for another take on the Philly cheesesteak, or it tastes good cold too.

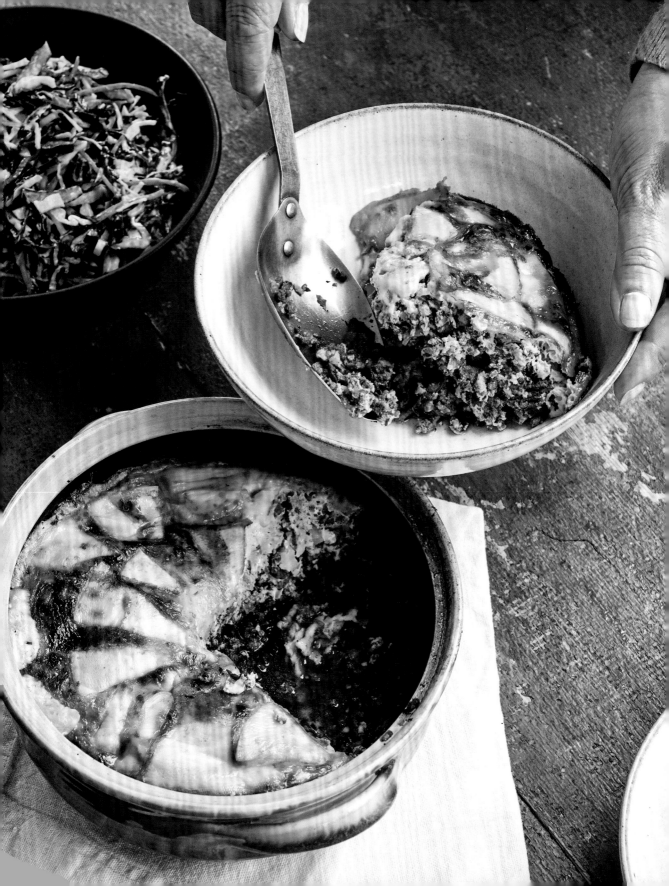

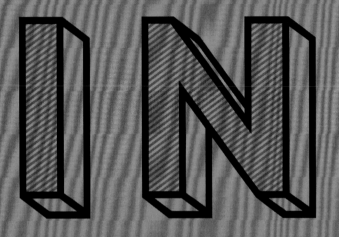 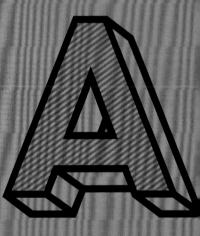

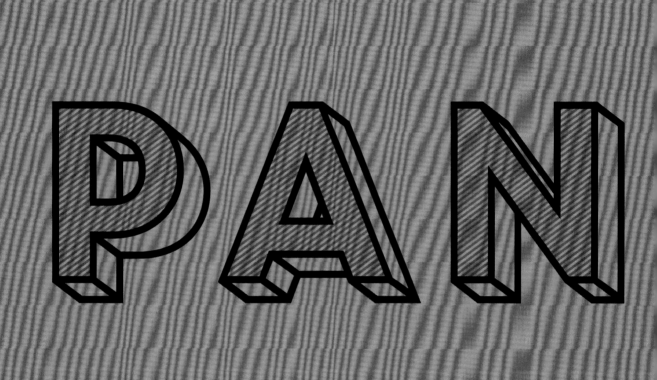

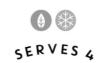

CHAPTER 2

VEGGIE JAMBALAYA

Originating in South Louisiana, jambalaya traditionally contains smoked sausage and often chicken and seafood, too. For this veggie version, the smokiness comes from smoked paprika, while I've used black-eyed beans for protein. I've also used brown rice for added fibre, plus it holds up much better than white when reheating any leftovers.

CALORIES PER SERVING: 294
PREP TIME: 15 MINUTES
COOK TIME: 40 MINUTES

spray oil
1 onion, finely chopped
2 celery sticks, finely chopped
2 peppers (1 red and 1 green), deseeded and finely chopped
1 carrot, peeled and very finely chopped
1 green chilli, deseeded and finely chopped
2 teaspoons dried oregano
½ teaspoon dried thyme
2 teaspoons smoked paprika
½ teaspoon ground turmeric
½ teaspoon cayenne pepper
1 teaspoon salt
½ teaspoon pepper
2 garlic cloves, crushed
150g (5½oz) brown basmati rice
750ml (1 pint 7fl oz) hot vegetable stock, plus extra if needed
400g (14oz) can of chopped tomatoes
400g (14oz) can of black-eyed beans, drained and rinsed
2 bay leaves
large handful of parsley leaves, finely chopped, plus extra to serve

1. Spray a sauté pan (with a lid) with oil and fry the onion, celery, peppers, carrot and chilli for 8 minutes, stirring occasionally.
2. Stir in the herbs and spices, salt and pepper, then add the garlic. Stir the rice through and then pour in the hot stock and tomatoes and add the black-eyed beans.
3. Add the bay leaves, cover the pan and simmer for 25 minutes, stirring every now and again.
4. Remove the lid, stir through the chopped parsley and simmer for another 5 minutes to bubble away any excess liquid.
5. Check the rice is cooked (if not, allow it to simmer for longer, adding more stock if necessary), then serve with parsley scattered over the top.

NOTE If you want to add smoky sausage or chicken to this, fry it with the vegetables in step 1. Seafood such as cooked prawns can be added for the last 10 minutes of simmering. Leftovers are great served with a fried egg.

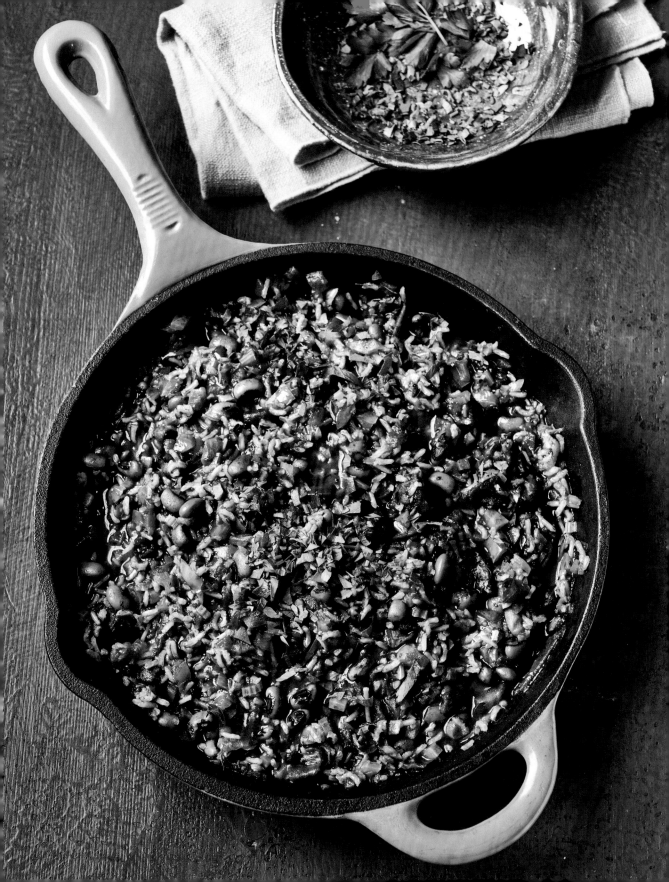

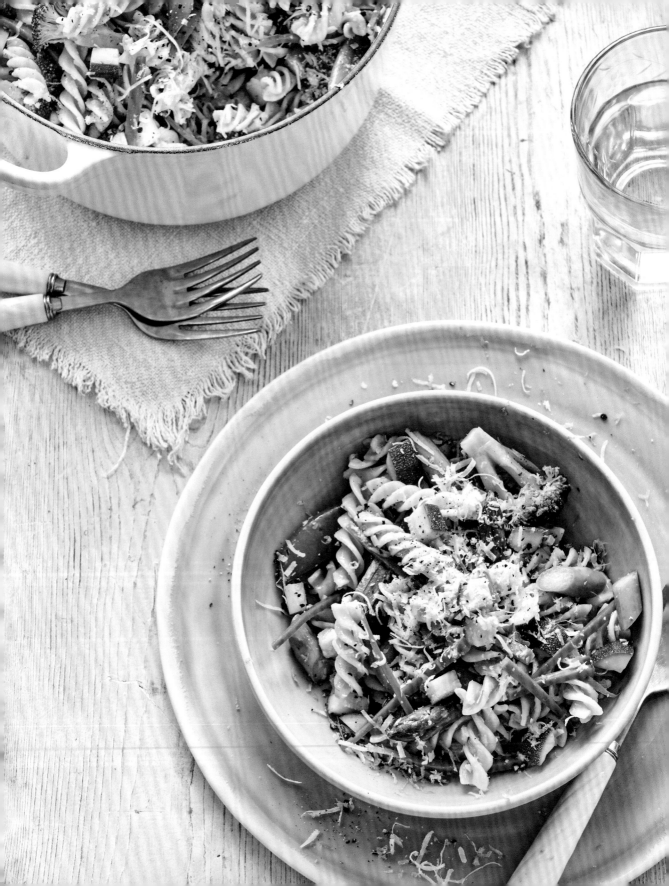

SPRING-ON-A-PLATE FUSILLI

The lightest of pasta dishes with a hint of lemon and garlic and plenty of fresh, al dente vegetables. This is a great sharing dish for spring and summer, or a vitamin boost for the winter months.

CALORIES PER SERVING: 288
PREP TIME: 20 MINUTES
COOK TIME: 15 MINUTES

1 teaspoon unsalted butter
1 shallot, very finely chopped
2 garlic cloves, crushed
1 teaspoon coarse sea salt
250g (9oz) fusilli pasta
750ml (1 pint 7fl oz) boiling water
6 asparagus spears, woody ends trimmed away, sliced diagonally into 1cm (½ inch) pieces
1 small courgette, finely chopped
1 carrot, peeled and julienned, or cut into very fine batons
½ head of broccoli, broken into small florets
80g (2¾oz) sugarsnap peas, halved on the diagonal
30g (1oz) Parmesan-style vegetarian cheese, grated
finely grated zest of 1 unwaxed lemon
handful of basil leaves
pepper

1. Melt the butter in a large saucepan (with a lid) and add the shallot, garlic and coarse sea salt. Stir-fry over a gentle heat for 2 minutes.
2. Add the fusilli and measured boiling water, bring to the boil, then simmer for 8 minutes, stirring a couple of times during this time.
3. Add all the prepared vegetables. Place the lid on the pan and simmer for 3 minutes.
4. Remove the lid and check the pasta is cooked (if not, place the lid back on and cook for 5 more minutes before checking again). Stir in most of the cheese and half the lemon zest (there is no need to drain the pan beforehand).
5. Serve immediately, scattered with the remaining cheese and lemon zest and a few grinds of black pepper, and garnished with torn basil leaves.

NOTE This is the perfect dish to use up fresh seasonal vegetables. You could add broad beans, runner beans, green beans, peas, spinach, spring onions or marrow. If you have fresh salad leaves, such as rocket or watercress, you could garnish the finished plates of pasta with a handful. If you like a bit of spice, then fry a finely chopped red chilli with the shallot in step 1.

BLACK BEAN & MUSHROOM DAL

This is a long-standing family favourite for us, as my mum and I learned how to cook it at an Indian cookery evening run by another parent at my secondary school in the 1990s! I wish I could credit her, but sadly my memory is not good enough to remember her name. We have cooked this so many times over the years and the only change I have made is to use canned black-eyed beans instead of dried. It is a very quick dish to pull together, so it's great for a quick and easy lunch, and is full of flavour and texture. It can be eaten as a stand-alone meal or is a great vegetarian dish to serve alongside curries for an Indian spread.

CALORIES PER SERVING: 122
PREP TIME: 5 MINUTES
COOK TIME: 25 MINUTES

spray oil
1 onion, finely chopped
½ teaspoon cumin seeds
½ teaspoon pepper
½ teaspoon garam masala
200g (7oz) mushrooms, sliced
400g (14oz) can of chopped tomatoes
400g (14oz) can of black-eyed beans, drained and rinsed
1 green chilli, deseeded and finely chopped
salt

TO SERVE
coriander leaves
lemon wedges

1. Spray a sauté pan or deep frying pan with oil and fry the onion for 5 minutes, then add the cumin seeds, pepper, garam masala and mushrooms and stir-fry for 5 minutes.
2. Add the tomatoes, black-eyed beans and chilli and simmer for 15 minutes. The curry should have quite a dry consistency.
3. Season to taste with salt and serve scattered with coriander leaves and with lemon wedges on the side.

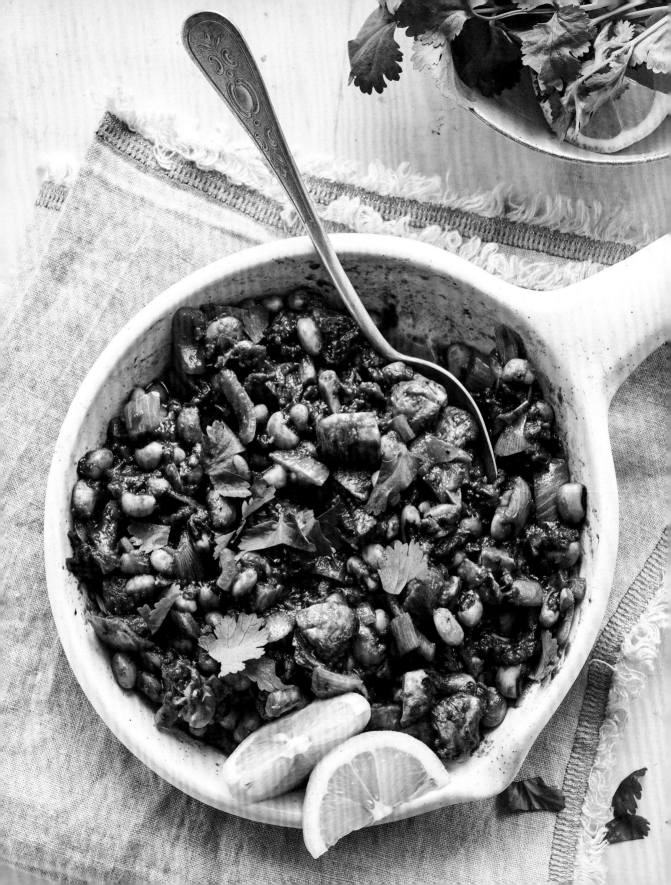

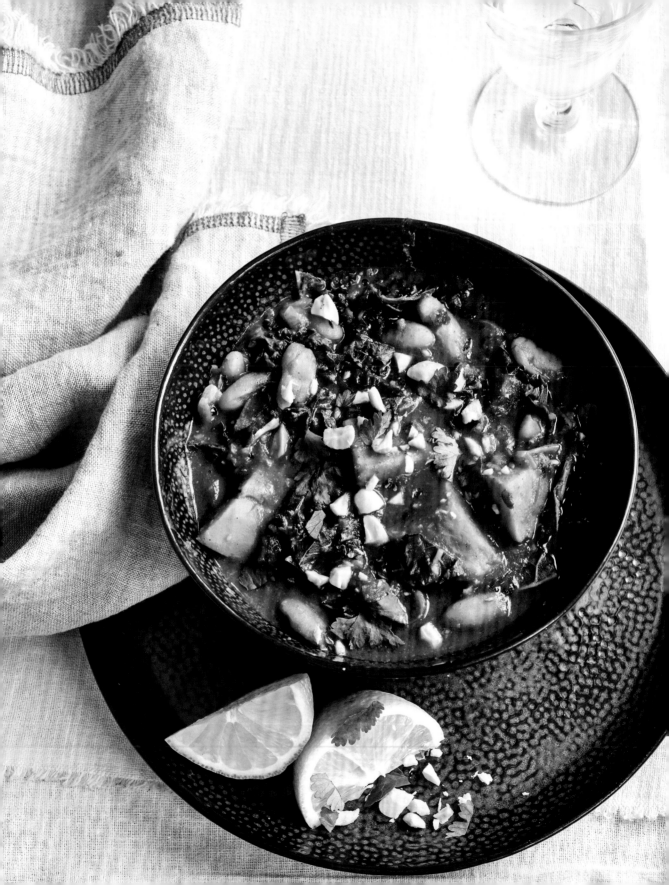

SPICY PEANUT STEW

Inspired by West African peanut stews, this vegan version has a thick and rich sauce encasing hearty sweet potato and beans. I serve this up in a bowl on its own, but if you prefer you can serve it with rice or bread.

CALORIES PER SERVING: 309
PREP TIME: 10 MINUTES
COOK TIME: 40 MINUTES

spray oil
1 onion, finely chopped
4 garlic cloves, crushed
3cm (1¼ inch) piece of fresh
 root ginger, peeled and grated
1 teaspoon smoked paprika
1 teaspoon ground cumin
1 teaspoon chilli flakes
½ teaspoon ground cinnamon
1 teaspoon dried thyme
3 tablespoons tomato purée
400g (14oz) can of chopped
 tomatoes
1 litre (1¾ pints) hot vegetable
 stock
1 large sweet potato (total
 weight about 500g/1lb 2oz),
 peeled and finely chopped
400g (14oz) can of cannellini
 beans, drained and rinsed
3 tablespoons smooth peanut
 butter
100g (3½oz) kale, roughly
 chopped
salt and pepper

TO SERVE
coriander leaves
lemon wedges
crushed peanuts (optional)

1. Spray a large saucepan with oil and fry the onion for 5 minutes.
2. Add the garlic and ginger and stir-fry for 30 seconds, then add the spices and thyme and stir them in, frying gently for another 30 seconds. Squeeze in the tomato purée and mix it in to form a paste with the other ingredients.
3. Add the chopped tomatoes, hot stock, sweet potato, cannellini beans and peanut butter. Give all the ingredients a thorough mix, then simmer the stew for 30 minutes.
4. Season with salt and pepper, stir in the kale and simmer for another 3 minutes.
5. Serve with coriander leaves and lemon wedges, and scatter over some crushed peanuts, if you like.

NOTE I have just used 1 teaspoon of chilli flakes here for convenience. But if you have access to scotch bonnet chillies, you can add a delicious fruity and authentic heat. Scotch bonnets are very hot indeed... I would probably only use half of one in this, but you know how spicy you like it!

CREAMED CORN CHOWDER PILAF

This is a great, simple vegetarian rice dish with mild flavours and a satisfying juxtaposition of consistency between soft rice and crunchy corn. This can be eaten as a stand-alone meal, but also makes a great side dish to grilled or barbecued meats such as sausages or peri-peri chicken.

CALORIES PER SERVING: 400
PREP TIME: 5 MINUTES
COOK TIME: 30 MINUTES

1 teaspoon unsalted butter
1 onion, finely chopped
1 garlic clove, crushed
600g (1lb 5oz) frozen sweetcorn, defrosted
1 litre (1¾ pints) hot vegetable stock, plus extra if needed
100ml (3½fl oz) semi-skimmed milk
250g (9oz) long grain rice
100g (3½oz) light cream cheese
pepper
parsley leaves, to serve

FOR THE SPICE MIX
1 teaspoon smoked paprika
1 teaspoon dried thyme
1 teaspoon salt
½ teaspoon pepper
½ teaspoon onion granules
½ teaspoon garlic granules

1. Mix together all the ingredients for the spice mix.
2. Using a sauté pan (with a lid), melt the butter and fry the onion for 5 minutes until soft. Add the garlic, sweetcorn and spice mix, stir together, then pour in about half the hot stock and all the milk. Bring up to a simmer and simmer for 5 minutes.
3. Using a ladle, remove 2 ladlefuls of the mixture and place in a bowl. Use a hand blender or mini chopper to purée it, then return it to the sauté pan. (This will add to the creamy consistency and yellow colour of the final dish.)
4. Add the rice and remaining stock to the pan, stir it through and place the lid on. Simmer gently for 15 minutes. Remove the lid from the pan, stir, then allow it to bubble for 5 minutes with the lid off.
5. Check that the rice is cooked (if not, allow it to simmer for longer, adding more stock if necessary), then stir through the cream cheese.
6. Season with black pepper and serve scattered with finely chopped parsley.

NOTE A very tasty addition to this (for non-vegetarians) is some chopped smoked bacon or chorizo. If you are adding either of these, fry them along with the onion in step 2. If you are using bacon with fat, or chorizo, then there is no need to use the butter.

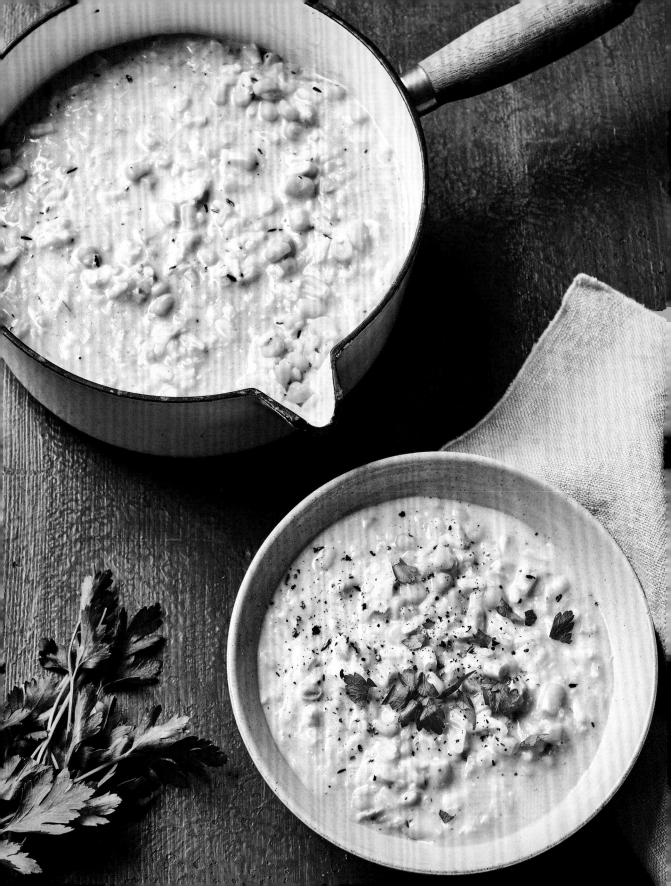

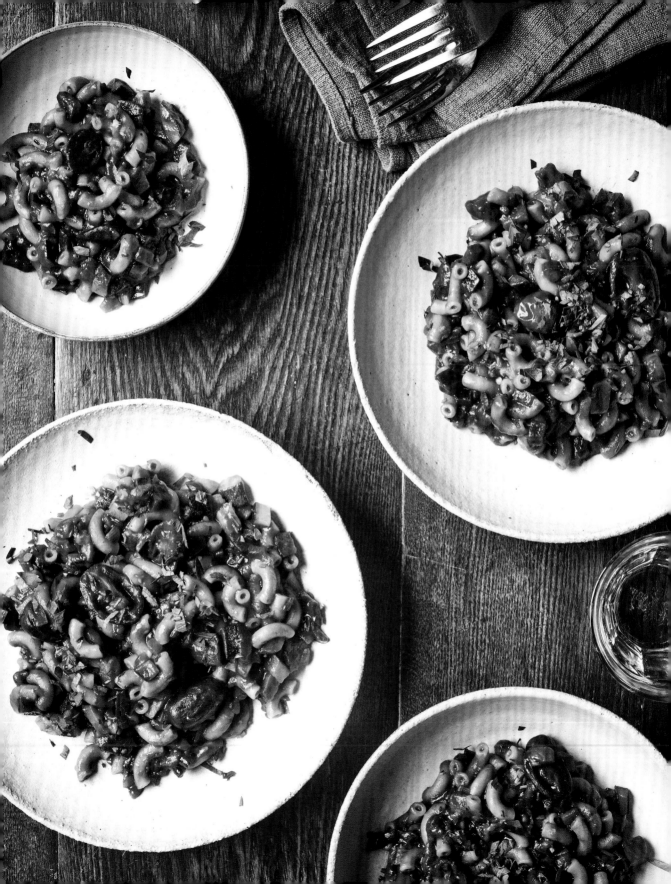

MAC'A'RATATOUILLE

All the delicious flavours of ratatouille in an all-in-one macaroni dish. I like to chop the veg really small for this, so it really complements the macaroni, and it's a great way to introduce fussier kids to these vegetables. You might not be able to resist smothering this in cheese and finishing it off under the grill, but it is delicious just as it is.

CALORIES PER SERVING: 361
PREP TIME: 15 MINUTES
COOK TIME: 35 MINUTES

1 teaspoon olive oil
1 red onion, finely chopped
1 aubergine, finely chopped
1 courgette, finely chopped
1 red pepper, deseeded and finely
   chopped
200g (7oz) cherry tomatoes,
   halved
2 garlic cloves, crushed
1 teaspoon coarse sea salt
1 tablespoon balsamic vinegar
500ml (18fl oz) tomato passata
700ml (1¼ pints) hot vegetable
   stock
250g (9oz) macaroni
1 teaspoon dried thyme
1 teaspoon dried rosemary
pepper
chopped parsley leaves, to serve

1. Put the oil in a deep nonstick saucepan, turn the heat to high and add the onion, aubergine, courgette, pepper, cherry tomatoes, garlic and salt and fry for 10 minutes, stirring regularly to prevent burning and sticking. Stir in the balsamic vinegar.
2. Stir in the passata, hot stock, macaroni, thyme and rosemary and cook on a fast simmer for 25 minutes. Stir regularly to stop the macaroni from sticking to the bottom of the pan.
3. After 25 minutes, the macaroni should be cooked through (if not, cook for 5 more minutes before checking again) and the sauce should be thick and rich. If the sauce looks too watery, give it a couple more minutes bubbling away at a high heat.
4. Scatter with parsley and serve immediately.

NOTE If you'd like to add meat to this meal, chorizo, bacon or sausage all work really well: just chop them up and fry them with the vegetables in step 1.

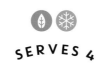

PANEER & SPINACH TIKKA MASALA

Lentils, spinach and cubes of paneer in a rich tikka masala sauce. Paneer is an Indian cheese with a mild flavour and firm consistency which allows it to hold up well in a sauce without melting, and is great at absorbing flavours. You can enjoy a bowl of this as a stand-alone meal or serve it up with naan or wholemeal pitta.

CALORIES PER SERVING: 332
PREP TIME: 15 MINUTES, PLUS
2–3 MINUTES STANDING
COOK TIME: 25 MINUTES

spray oil
200g (7oz) paneer, chopped into
   1cm (½ inch) cubes
1 onion, finely chopped
1 red pepper, deseeded and finely
   chopped
400g (14oz) can of chopped
   tomatoes
400g (14oz) can of green lentils,
   drained and rinsed
200ml (7fl oz) boiling water
150g (5½oz) baby spinach
150g (5½oz) fat-free Greek yogurt
salt and pepper
coriander leaves, to serve

FOR THE CURRY PASTE
4 garlic cloves
3cm (1¼ inch) piece of fresh root
   ginger, peeled
1 red chilli, deseeded
1 teaspoon ground turmeric
2 tablespoons tomato purée
1 tablespoon garam masala
2 tablespoons water

1. Spray a sauté pan with oil and fry the paneer cubes for 3–4 minutes until the edges are starting to go golden brown. Scoop the paneer from the pan and set aside in a bowl.

2. Make up the curry paste: place all the ingredients into a mini chopper and whizz into a smooth paste.

3. Fry the onion in the sauté pan, in more spray oil if needed, for 5 minutes, then add the curry paste: stir-fry gently for 2 minutes until you can smell the spices, but be careful not to burn the paste. Stir in the pepper, then the chopped tomatoes, green lentils and measured boiling water. Stir thoroughly and simmer over a medium heat for 15 minutes.

4. Stir the spinach into the sauce, remove from the heat, then spoon the yogurt on top. Leave it sitting on top of the sauce for 2 minutes before stirring it through; this allows it to warm through and lessens the chance of it splitting.

5. Return the paneer to the curry, season to taste and serve scattered with coriander leaves.

NOTE You can substitute the paneer for extra vegetables – cubes of aubergine, butternut squash or sweet potato all work well – fried with the onion in step 3, allowing them longer to simmer in step 5 (about 30 minutes).

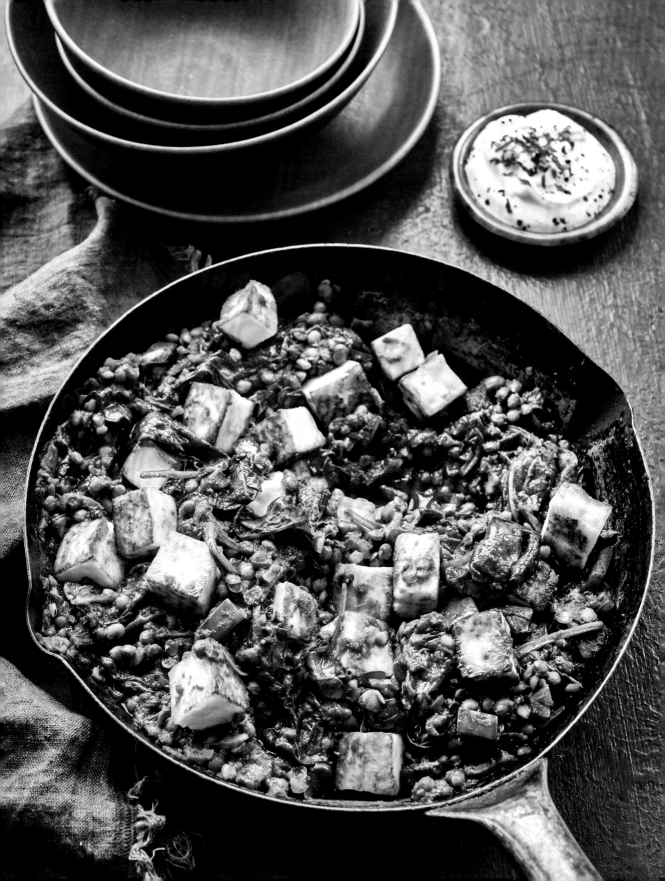

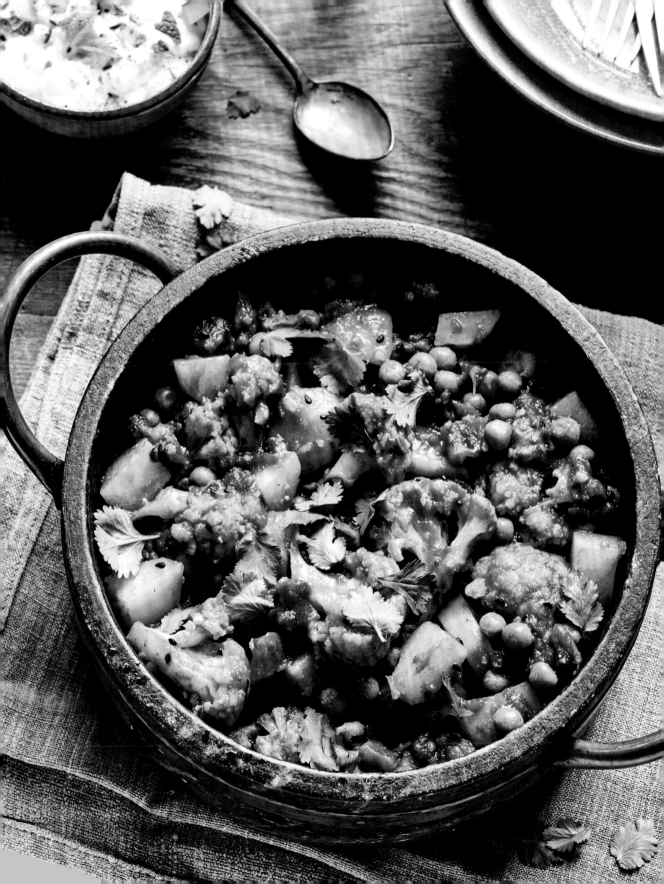

CAULIFLOWER, POTATO & PEA CURRY

A meat-free curry that is light but satisfying. A great stand-alone dish with no need for rice, but which also works well with a mix of other dishes for a family curry night.

CALORIES PER SERVING: 227
PREP TIME: 10 MINUTES
COOK TIME: 25 MINUTES

spray oil
about 500g (1lb 2oz) potatoes, peeled and cut into bite-sized chunks
1 medium cauliflower, cut into same-sized florets
400g (14oz) can of chopped tomatoes
large handful of coriander leaves, chopped, plus extra to serve
250ml (9fl oz) boiling water
1 teaspoon salt
200g (7oz) frozen peas, defrosted
juice of 1 lemon

FOR THE SPICE MIX
1 teaspoon mustard seeds
1 teaspoon ground cumin
1 teaspoon nigella seeds
½ teaspoon ground turmeric
½ teaspoon chilli flakes

1. Make up the spice mix by mixing all the ingredients together in a small bowl.
2. Spray a sauté pan (with a lid) with oil and stir-fry the potatoes and cauliflower for 5 minutes. Add the spice mix and stir-fry for another minute.
3. Add the tomatoes, coriander, measured boiling water and salt, place the lid on the pan and leave to simmer for 15 minutes.
4. Stir in the peas, squeeze in the lemon juice and cook over a high heat for 3 minutes, giving the sauce a good bubble and allowing it to reduce and thicken. Garnish with some more coriander and serve.

CUCUMBER & MINT RAITA
Make a quick cucumber and mint raita to go with this, or any other curry. Raita has a sweet and fresh flavour and makes a cooling side dish. Just combine 250g (9oz) fat-free Greek yogurt, 2 crushed garlic cloves, a handful of mint leaves (very finely chopped), one-quarter of a cucumber (very finely chopped), a couple of pinches of salt and ½ teaspoon of garam masala. Mix everything together and serve in a small bowl alongside the curry.

MUSHROOM PESTO QUINOTTO

Quinoa is a great alternative to rice or couscous for a one-pot dish. It is a gluten-free whole grain which is high in fibre and protein, cooked here in a similar way to a risotto, adding more stock as you go until the grain is fully cooked. Red pesto and plenty of fresh basil add easy, great flavour to the finished dish.

CALORIES PER SERVING: 299
PREP TIME: 10 MINUTES,
PLUS STANDING TIME
COOK TIME: 30 MINUTES

spray oil
1 onion, finely chopped
300g (10½oz) chestnut
   mushrooms, sliced
2 garlic cloves, crushed
200g (7oz) quinoa
1 litre (1¾ pints) hot vegetable
   stock
175g (6oz) frozen petits pois,
   defrosted
1 large courgette, finely chopped
3 tablespoons red pesto
salt and pepper

TO SERVE
large handful of basil leaves
Parmesan cheese, grated
   (optional)

1. Spray a sauté pan or nonstick flameproof casserole dish (with a lid) with oil and fry the onion and mushrooms gently for 8 minutes. Add the garlic and stir through, then add the quinoa.

2. Pour 500ml (18fl oz) of the hot stock into the pan and allow to simmer gently for 10 minutes, stirring occasionally. Now pour in the remaining stock, bring up to a fast simmer and simmer for 5 minutes.

3. Add the peas and courgette, season with salt and pepper and simmer for 5 more minutes.

4. Remove from the heat and stir through the pesto. Place the lid on the pan and leave to stand for 5 minutes.

5. Serve with plenty of basil leaves and cheese, if you like.

NOTE If you would like to make this dish vegetarian, look out for a vegetarian red pesto (many contain non-vegetarian cheese), as well as a Parmesan-style vegetarian cheese to grate over the top.

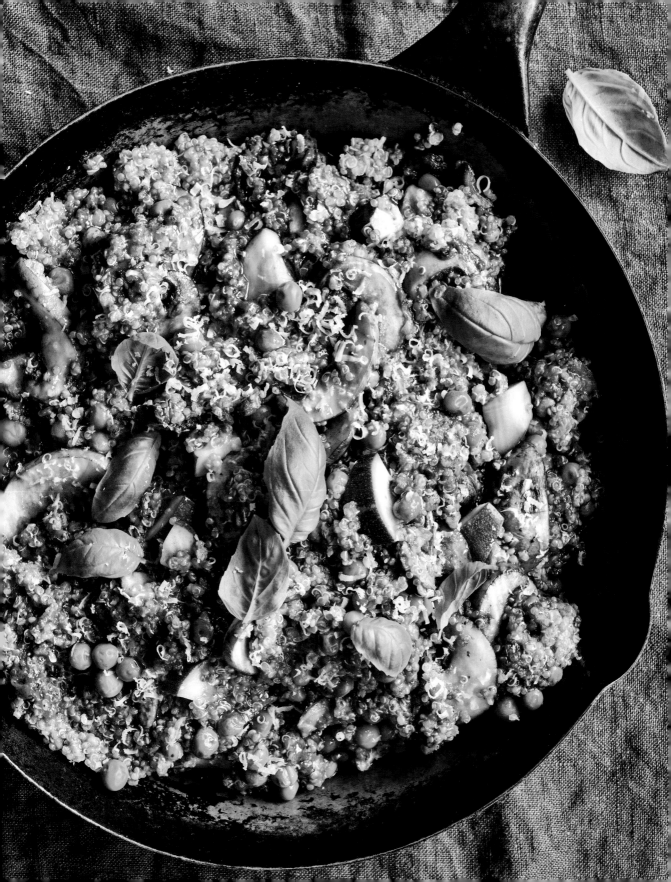

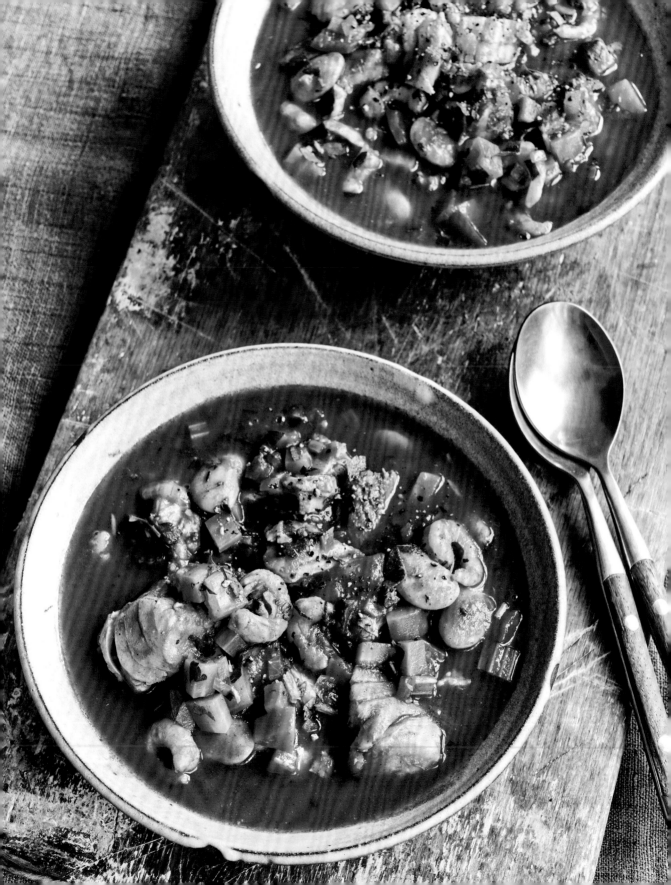

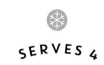

SHIPWRECK CHOWDER

A hearty and flavoursome fish stew swimming with tender, flaky white fish, such as haddock cod or basa, nutritious sardines, prawns and creamy butter beans, all in a rich tomato sauce.

CALORIES PER PORTION: 368
PREP TIME: 15 MINUTES
COOK TIME: 1 HOUR 10 MINUTES

spray oil
1 onion, finely chopped
2 celery sticks, finely chopped
2 carrots, peeled and finely
    chopped
1 red pepper, deseeded and very
    finely chopped
4 garlic cloves, crushed
750ml (1 pint 7fl oz) hot fish stock
500ml (18fl oz) tomato passata
1 teaspoon sweet paprika
½ teaspoon cayenne pepper
¼ teaspoon ground cinnamon
1 teaspoon salt
½ teaspoon dried thyme
3 tablespoons Worcestershire sauce
3 tablespoons tomato purée
large handful of parsley leaves,
    chopped, plus extra to serve
300g (10½oz) white fish fillets,
    chopped small
120g (4¼oz) can of sardines in
    tomato sauce
400g (14oz) can of butter beans,
    drained and rinsed
2 bay leaves
200g (7oz) cooked and peeled
    cold-water prawns
juice of 1 lemon
pepper

1. Spray a large flameproof casserole dish with oil and fry the onion, celery, carrots, pepper and garlic for 10 minutes over a gentle heat.
2. Pour in the hot stock and add the passata, spices, salt and thyme, Worcestershire sauce, tomato purée and parsley and stir everything together. Add the white fish, sardines (break these apart a bit with a fork as you add them) and butter beans.
3. Pop the bay leaves into the pan and leave simmering gently for 1 hour, uncovered.
4. When there is 10 minutes of cooking time remaining, add the prawns and lemon juice, then simmer for the final 10 minutes.
5. Serve in bowls with grindings of pepper and scattered with parsley. (Make sure to fish out the bay leaves.)

NOTE I've added sardines to this as they are a great oily fish, they add fantastic flavour and are excellent value, so this stew doesn't need lots of super-expensive fresh fish. You can customize it to your own tastes: replace the white fish with salmon fillets, or add other favourite seafood such as calamari and mussels, just double-check how long they should cook for and throw them in the pot at the right time! To take any spiciness out, omit the cayenne pepper, or for a bit more spice, a finely chopped red chilli can be added in step 1.

SPICY PRAWN ARROZ

Peppery prawns with garlic and a hint of lemon add amazing flavour to this Spanish-inspired rice dish.

CALORIES PER SERVING: 371
PREP TIME: 10 MINUTES
COOK TIME: 30 MINUTES

spray oil
300g (10½oz) cooked and peeled cold-water prawns (if frozen, ensure they are thoroughly defrosted)
2 red chillies, deseeded and finely chopped
3 garlic cloves, crushed
1 unwaxed lemon, zested, then cut into wedges
¼ teaspoon pepper
1 onion, finely chopped
2 tablespoons red wine vinegar
1 red pepper, deseeded and finely chopped
1 green pepper, deseeded and finely chopped
300g (10½oz) basmati rice
800ml (1 pint 9fl oz) hot vegetable stock
2 tablespoons tomato purée
salt
small handful of parsley leaves, chopped to serve

1. Spray a sauté pan, shallow flameproof casserole dish or large, deep frying pan with oil, bring up to a high heat and add the prawns, chillies, garlic, lemon zest and pepper. Stir-fry for 2 minutes, then set aside in a bowl.
2. Spray a little more oil into the pan, add the onion and vinegar and stir-fry for 3 minutes. Add the peppers and fry for 3 minutes.
3. Stir the rice in, then pour in 600ml (20fl oz) of the hot stock, add the tomato purée, bring up to a fast simmer and simmer for 15 minutes, stirring occasionally. (If the rice starts to dry out too much during the cooking time, add a little more of the stock to keep it cooking and prevent it from burning.) Return the prawn mixture, stirring it through the rice and allow to simmer for 5 minutes. Season with salt.
4. Try a little of the rice to check it is cooked through (if not, allow it to simmer for longer, adding more stock if necessary).
5. Serve with chopped parsley and lemon wedges.

NOTE If you'd like to make this vegetarian, you can replace the prawns with some extra vegetables, such as mushrooms. Just start the dish at step 2 with the chillies, garlic, lemon zest, pepper, then add the new vegetables with the peppers.

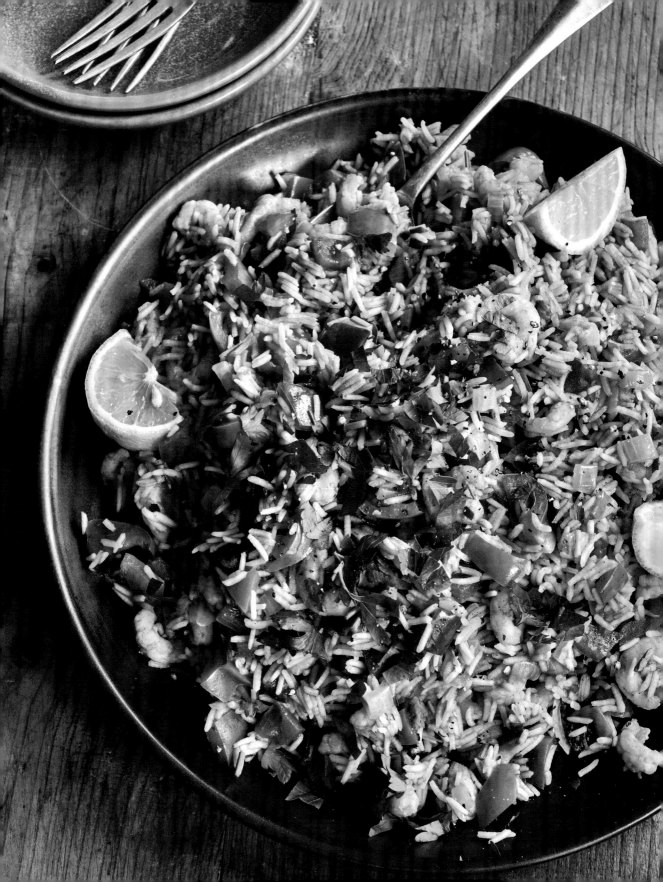

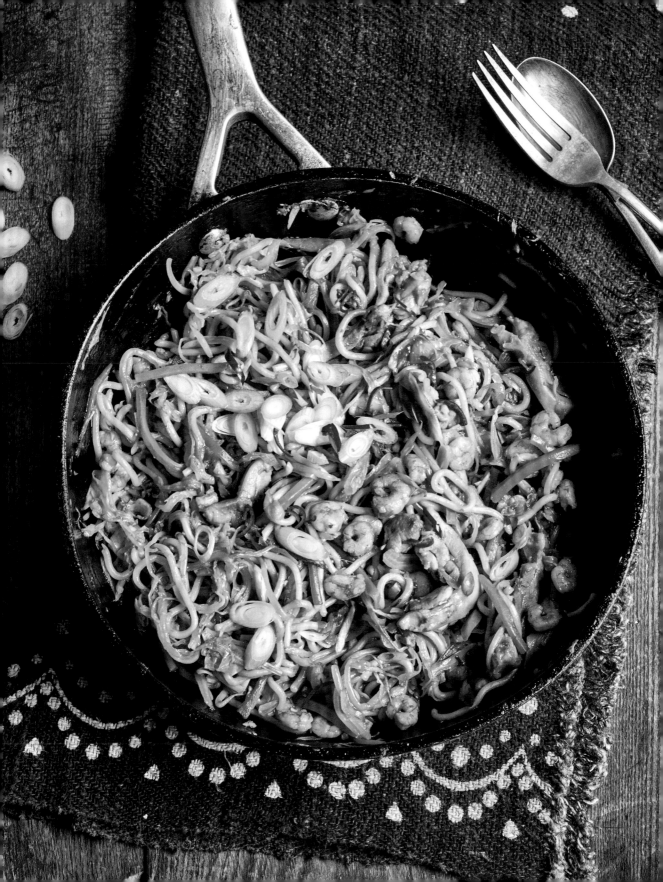

SPECIAL CHOW MEIN

This was always my dish of choice from the Chinese takeaway: I love its mix of spicy noodles, variety of crunchy vegetables and different meats or seafood. I've used my favourite combination of chicken and prawns here. There's a little cheat in this recipe, with ready-cooked noodles making it a true one-pan meal, but of course if you prefer you can cook your own noodles to add in.

CALORIES PER SERVING: 580
PREP TIME: 15 MINUTES
COOK TIME: 10 MINUTES

3 garlic cloves, crushed

3 spring onions, cut into matchsticks, plus extra, sliced, to serve

1 birds' eye chilli, deseeded and finely chopped

¼ white cabbage, very finely sliced

1 large carrot, peeled and cut into thin matchsticks

1 teaspoon sesame oil

2 chicken thigh fillets, excess fat removed, finely sliced

150g (5½oz) cooked and peeled cold-water prawns

300g (10½oz) straight-to-wok medium noodles

2 large handfuls of beansprouts

FOR THE CHOW MEIN SAUCE

2 tablespoons light soy sauce

3 tablespoons oyster sauce

1 tablespoon Shaoxing rice wine

1. Prepare the sauce in a small bowl by mixing together the soy sauce, oyster sauce and rice wine.

2. To be quick when you start cooking (as you want everything to be perfectly cooked to keep the vegetables crunchy), prepare the garlic, spring onions, chilli, cabbage and carrot, and put them all into one bowl, ready to tip into the pan when you need them.

3. In a sauté pan or wok, heat the sesame oil and stir-fry the chicken for 2 minutes over a high heat. Add the prepared vegetable mix and stir-fry this for 4 minutes, keeping the heat high. Tip in the prawns and stir-fry for 2 more minutes.

4. Next, add the noodles, loosen them up so that you can stir-fry them, add the beansprouts and stir-fry everything for 2 minutes.

5. Finally, pour in the sauce, spend 30 seconds stirring it in to coat all the ingredients, then serve straightaway, scattered with sliced spring onions.

NOTE This is a great dish for using up leftover roast meat such as pork, chicken or beef. Just cut it into fine slices and add it with the vegetables in step 3, so it has a chance to heat through properly.

SWEET & SOUR RICE POT

A family favourite, sweet and sour chicken, made into an all-in-one dish with fluffy rice and crunchy water chestnuts. This is a mild-flavoured dish and is great on its own, or served as part of a homemade Chinese feast.

CALORIES PER SERVING: 479
PREP TIME: 15 MINUTES, PLUS STANDING TIME
COOK TIME: 25 MINUTES

spray oil
1 onion, finely chopped
3 skinless chicken breasts (total weight about 500g/1lb 2oz), finely chopped
1 red pepper, deseeded and very finely chopped
2 garlic cloves, crushed
300g (10½oz) long grain white rice
2 canned pineapple rings (total weight about 65g/2½oz), very finely chopped
100g (3½oz) Tenderstem broccoli, sliced into 2cm (¾ inch) lengths
225g (8oz) can of water chestnuts, drained
800ml (1 pint 9fl oz) hot chicken stock, plus extra if needed
salt and pepper

FOR THE SAUCE
2 tablespoons tomato ketchup
2 tablespoons white rice vinegar
1 tablespoon light soy sauce
2 teaspoons light brown sugar

TO SERVE
spring onions, finely chopped
red chilli, finely chopped

1. Mix together all the ingredients for the sauce in a small bowl.
2. Spray a deep, nonstick flameproof casserole dish (with a lid) with oil (mine was 24cm/9½ inches in diameter). Fry the onion and chicken for 8 minutes. Season the dish, then add the pepper, garlic and sweet and sour sauce. Stir in the rice, then add the pineapple, broccoli, water chestnuts and hot stock.
3. Place the lid on the pan, and gently simmer for 15 minutes.
4. Remove the lid from the pan and simmer with the lid off for 2 minutes. Check that the rice is fully cooked (if not, allow it to simmer for longer, adding more stock if necessary).
5. Place the lid back on, remove the pan from the heat and leave to stand for 5 minutes. Serve scattered with spring onions and chilli.

NOTE You can always double up on the batch of sweet and sour sauce and reserve half to drizzle over the rice dish when you serve it. Just bring it to the boil in a small saucepan, add 2 tablespoons of water and let it simmer for a couple of minutes before serving up alongside the rice pot.

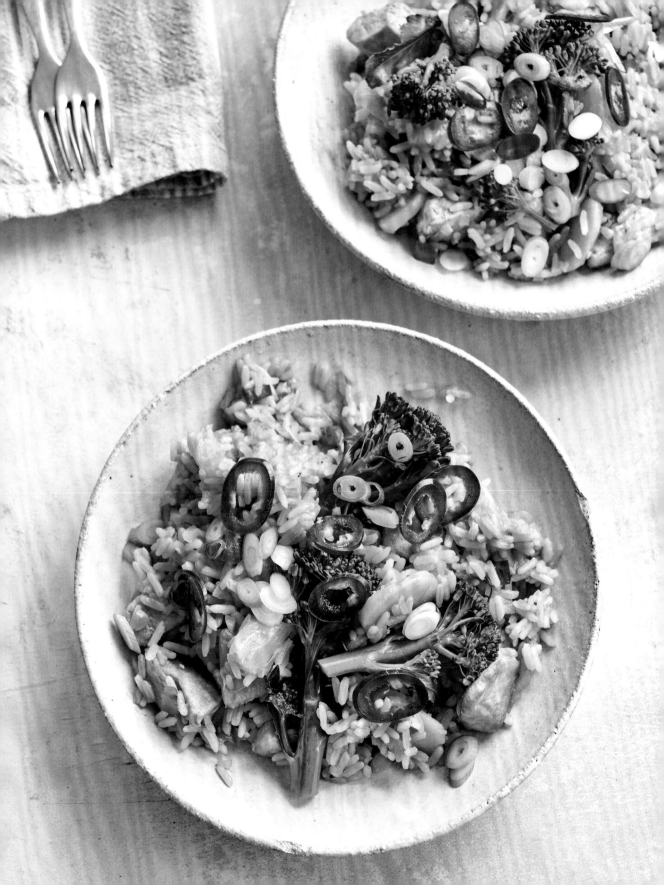

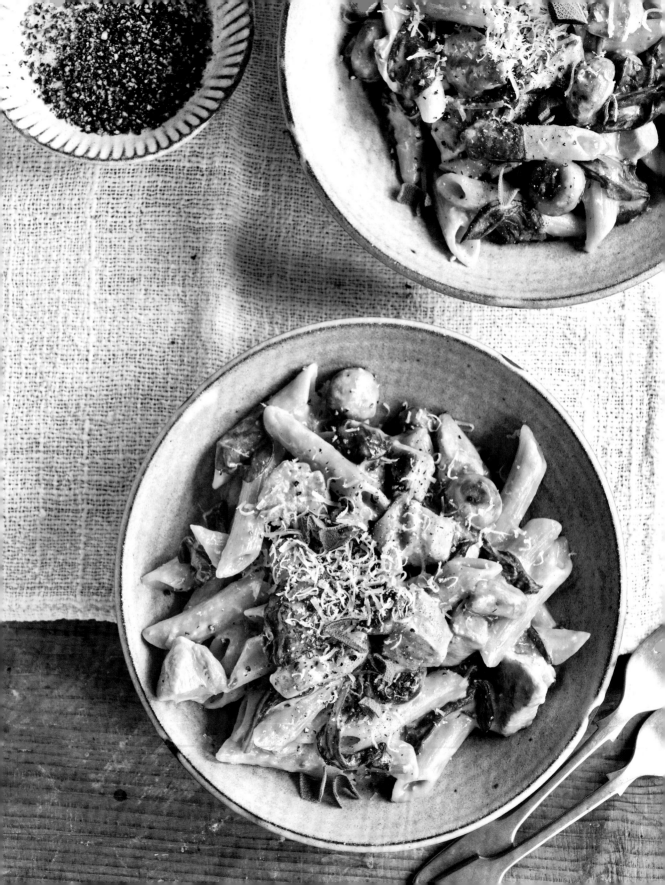

CREAMY CHICKEN, HONEY & MUSTARD PENNE

This is a throwback to university days for me. My friend Karen used to love a honey-mustard sauce when cooking chicken and the smell and taste of this takes me right back there! It is possible to achieve a creamy sauce without adding a lot of calories. I usually do it by adding milk to stock when I simmer the pasta, then stirring in either low-fat crème fraîche or light cream cheese at the end of cooking.

CALORIES PER SERVING: 548
PREP TIME: 10 MINUTES
COOK TIME: 20 MINUTES

spray oil
3–4 skinless chicken breasts
    (total weight about 600g/1lb
    5oz), chopped
3 garlic cloves, crushed
200g (7oz) button mushrooms
600ml (20fl oz) hot chicken
    stock
250ml (9fl oz) semi-skimmed
    milk
285g (10oz) penne
1 teaspoon cornflour
3 tablespoons half-fat crème
    fraîche
1 tablespoon honey
1 tablespoon Dijon mustard
2 large handfuls of baby spinach,
    roughly chopped
salt and pepper

TO SERVE
sage leaves, finely chopped
Parmesan cheese, grated

1. Spray a saucepan with oil and stir-fry the chicken for 3 minutes, then stir in the garlic and button mushrooms.
2. Pour in the hot stock and milk, bring to the boil and add the pasta. Simmer for 15 minutes, stirring occasionally.
3. In a small bowl, stir the cornflour into the crème fraîche.
4. Check that the pasta is cooked (if not, cook for 5 more minutes before checking again). Stir in the honey, mustard, crème fraîche mixture and baby spinach, then season with salt and pepper.
5. Serve with chopped sage and Parmesan on the top.

NOTE This also works as a vegetarian dish, just leave out the chicken, double the amount of mushrooms, swap the chicken stock for vegetable stock and use a Parmesan-style vegetarian cheese.

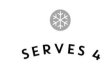

SERVES 4

LEMON CHICKEN
WITH MASALA CHICKPEAS

Tangy lemon and a fragrant masala curry paste give this curry amazing flavour. I use a sauté pan to make it, as it's great for frying and deep enough to hold all the ingredients while the curry simmers.

CALORIES PER SERVING: 415
PREP TIME: 15 MINUTES
(INCLUDING MAKING THE
CURRY PASTE)
COOK TIME: 40 MINUTES

juice of 2 lemons
3–4 skinless chicken breasts
    (total weight about 600g/1lb
    5oz), cut into chunks
½ teaspoon salt
spray oil
6 tablespoons Masala Curry
    Paste (see page 226)
400g (14oz) can of chopped
    tomatoes
400ml (14fl oz) boiling water
2 × 400g (14oz) cans of
    chickpeas, drained and rinsed
1 teaspoon garlic granules
1 tablespoon mango chutney
2 large handfuls of baby spinach

TO SERVE
nigella seeds
coriander leaves

1. In a small bowl, pour the lemon juice over the chicken chunks, add the salt and mix.
3. Spray a sauté pan with oil and stir-fry the chicken over a high heat for 5 minutes. Add the curry paste, stir in, then reduce the heat and gently sizzle the chicken and curry paste together for 2 minutes. Add the chopped tomatoes, measured boiling water, chickpeas and garlic granules. Stir well and bring up to a fast simmer.
4. Simmer the curry for 30 minutes, stirring occasionally.
5. Remove from the heat, then add the mango chutney and the spinach. Stir everything together until the spinach is wilted, then serve sprinkled with nigella seeds and coriander.

NOTE You can bulk this out with extra vegetables such as butternut squash, sweet potato, mushrooms, peppers or carrots, just add them in step 3 with the chopped tomatoes.

NO TIME TO MAKE A PASTE?
Chop 1 onion finely, crush 4 garlic cloves, grate 1 tablespoon of fresh root ginger and finely chop 2 green chillies. Fry these with the chicken in step 3. After 5 minutes, add a mix of 1 tablespoon ground cumin, 1 tablespoon ground coriander, 1 teaspoon chilli powder, 1 teaspoon ground turmeric, ½ teaspoon ground cinnamon, ½ teaspoon pepper and ½ teaspoon salt. Stir-fry with the chicken for 2 minutes, then add the chopped tomatoes in step 5 and follow the recipe above

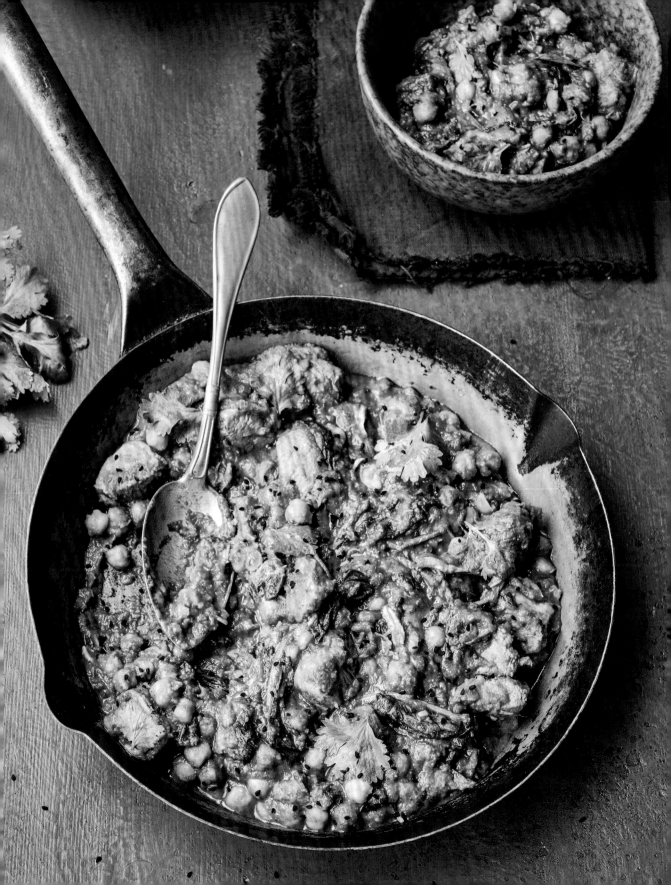

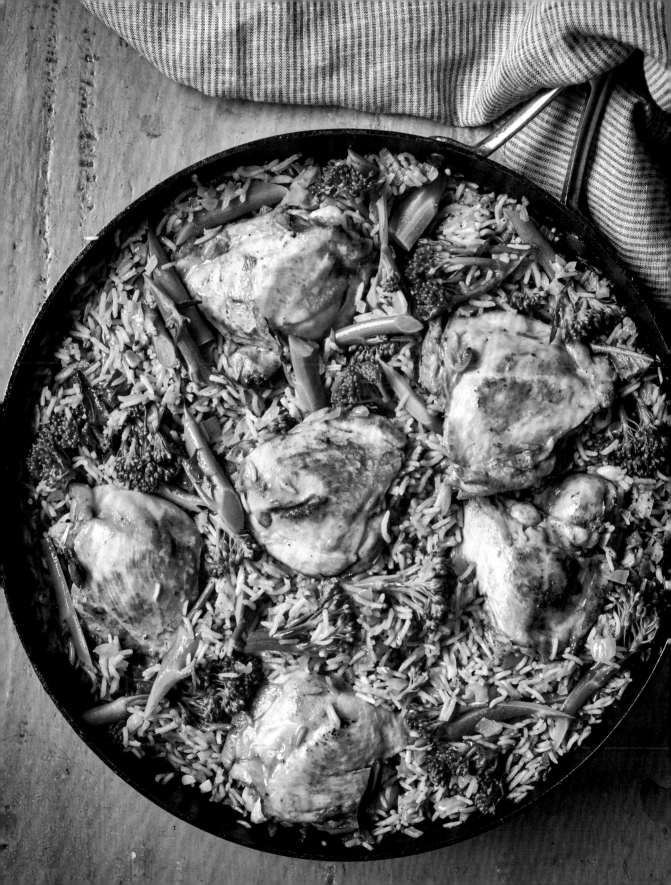

HOISIN CHICKEN & RICE
WITH TENDERSTEM BROCCOLI

This is a brilliant, easy stove-top supper. I use Tenderstem broccoli here, but you can add any favourite green vegetables such as green beans, sugarsnap peas or asparagus.

CALORIES PER SERVING: 493
PREP TIME: 15 MINUTES,
PLUS MARINATING TIME AND
RESTING TIME
COOK TIME: 20 MINUTES

6 chicken thigh fillets (total
   weight about 600g/1lb 5oz),
   fat trimmed and discarded
spray oil
1 onion, finely chopped
2 garlic cloves, crushed
1 tablespoon peeled and finely
   chopped fresh root ginger
200g (7oz) basmati rice
450ml (16fl oz) hot chicken stock
200g (7oz) Tenderstem broccoli,
   woody ends trimmed, cut into
   2cm (¾ inch) pieces

FOR THE MARINADE
2 garlic cloves, crushed
2 tablespoons Shaoxing rice wine
3 tablespoons hoisin sauce
2 tablespoons dark soy sauce
¼ teaspoon pepper

TO SERVE (OPTIONAL)
finely chopped red chilli
coriander leaves
chopped spring onions
cucumber ribbons or shavings

1. Put all the marinade ingredients into a large bowl, mix together and add the chicken thigh fillets, coating them thoroughly in the marinade. Allow to marinate for at least 10 minutes, or cover with clingfilm and leave for up to 1 day in the refrigerator.

2. Meanwhile, prepare and weigh out the other ingredients so they are all ready to use.

3. Spray a large, deep saucepan or flameproof pot (with a lid) with oil. Use tongs to lift the chicken from the marinade (reserve the marinade) and flash-fry the chicken over a high heat for 2 minutes on each side. Remove the chicken from the pan and set aside in a bowl.

4. Add the onion, garlic and ginger to the pan with a little extra spray oil and fry over a high heat for 1 minute. Add the rice to the pan, stir it in well, then pour in the hot stock, the reserved marinade and broccoli. Bring to a simmer, then place the chicken pieces on top of the rice.

5. Cover the pan with a lid and simmer over a medium heat for 15 minutes.

6. After 15 minutes, remove the pan from the heat (leaving the lid on) and allow to rest for 10 minutes. After this time the rice should be perfectly cooked.

7. Serve as it is, or with chopped red chilli, coriander leaves, chopped spring onions or cucumber ribbons if you like.

TURKEY TACO SPAGHETTI

This is such a satisfying spaghetti dish: tasty taco-filling flavours cooked with lean minced turkey, then coated in orange melted red Leicester cheese. A quick one-pot that really is more than the sum of its parts. I serve this with crunchy, shredded Little Gem lettuce, cherry tomatoes on the vine and lime wedges.

CALORIES PER SERVING: 404
PREP TIME: 10 MINUTES
COOK TIME: 20 MINUTES

spray oil
1 onion, finely chopped
250g (9oz) lean minced turkey
1 garlic clove, crushed
400g (14oz) can of chopped tomatoes
2 tablespoons finely chopped pickled jalapeños
450ml (16fl oz) water
250g (9oz) spaghetti, broken in half
60g (2¼oz) Red Leicester cheese, grated
salt and pepper
parsley leaves, chopped, to serve

FOR THE SPICE MIX
1 teaspoon garlic granules
1 teaspoon onion granules
1 teaspoon ground cumin
1 teaspoon dried oregano
1 teaspoon paprika (sweet, hot or smoked, to taste)

1. Mix together all the ingredients for the spice mix in a small bowl.

2. Spray a sauté pan (with a lid) with oil and fry the onion and minced turkey for 5 minutes, breaking down any clumps in the meat as it cooks (I use a wooden spoon for this).

3. Stir in the garlic and the spice mix, season with salt and pepper and stir-fry for 2 more minutes. Add the chopped tomatoes, jalapeños, measured water and spaghetti. Make sure all the pasta is submerged and give everything a good shuffle around to try and prevent the pasta from clumping.

4. Bring up to a simmer, pop the lid on the pan and allow to simmer without boiling over for 12 minutes (stir halfway through and nudge the spaghetti around to break up any bits that are sticking together).

5. Remove the lid, stir well and check that the spaghetti is cooked through and there are no uncooked clumps (if not, place the lid back on and cook for 5 more minutes before checking again). Stir the grated cheese through everything to coat the pasta and serve scattered with chopped parsley.

NOTE If you can't get hold of turkey, lean minced pork will also work well.

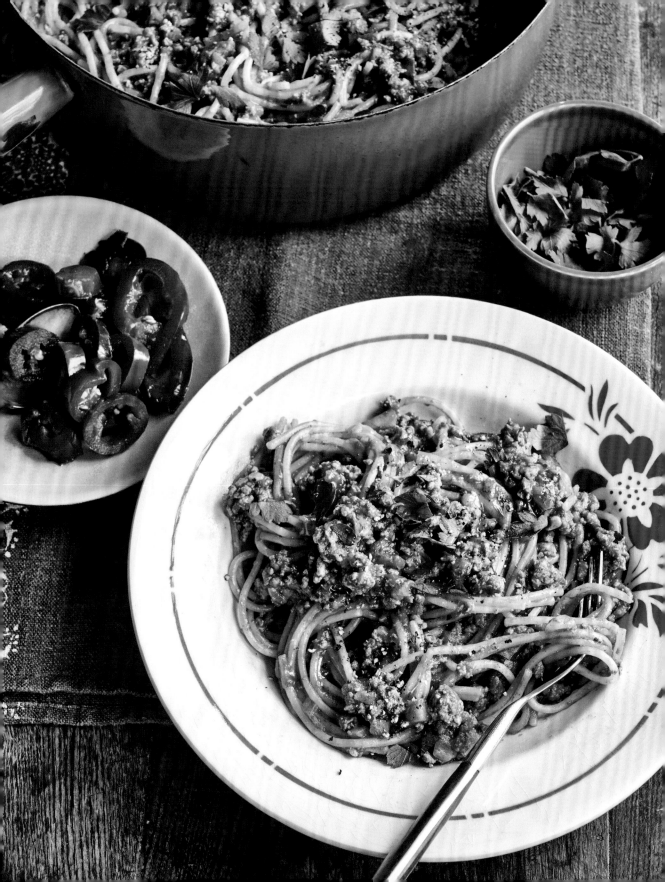

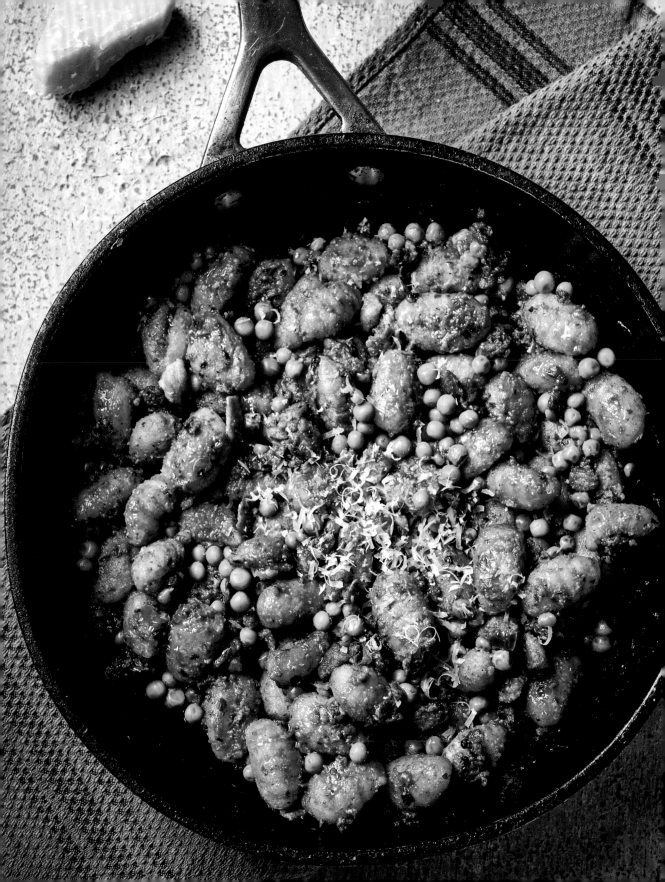

BACON GNOCCHI
WITH RED PESTO & PEAS

This is a midweek lifesaver: it has only a few ingredients – all easy to quickly pick up on a supermarket dash – and is ready in 15 minutes start-to-finish. Little pops of smoky bacon and peas complement the tender gnocchi. This amount of gnocchi does look like a small portion when plated up, but it is very filling and dense. I recommend serving it with salad (I usually have rocket or baby leaf salad with cherry tomatoes or chopped raw peppers) with my Crunchy Seed Sprinkle (see page 218) over the top or some freshly grated Parmesan cheese.

CALORIES PER SERVING: 262
PREP TIME: 5 MINUTES
COOK TIME: 10 MINUTES

1 teaspoon unsalted butter
4 smoked bacon medallions, finely chopped
4 shallots, finely chopped
500g (1lb 2oz) fresh gnocchi
1 garlic clove, crushed
100g (3½oz) frozen peas, defrosted
1 tablespoon red pesto
salt and pepper

1. In a frying pan, melt the butter and add the bacon, shallots, gnocchi and garlic. Stir-fry everything for 8 minutes over a medium heat. The gnocchi should turn golden brown.
2. Add the peas, season with salt and pepper and stir-fry for 2 more minutes.
3. Stir in the pesto and serve immediately.

NOTE This also works really well with chorizo instead of bacon, or green pesto in place of red. You can add extra green vegetables such as asparagus or green beans, cut into 2cm (¾ inch) pieces; fry them with the other ingredients in step 1.

RICH CHORIZO & ONION RIGATONI

A satisfyingly rich tomato sauce with fried onions, spicy tomato and fragrant chorizo. Chorizo and onions make a great combination to fry together: there is no need for extra oil and the onions take on a lovely colour and taste.

CALORIES PER SERVING: 381
PREP TIME: 10 MINUTES
COOK TIME: 45 MINUTES

50g (1¾oz) chorizo, very finely chopped
2 onions, finely sliced
250g (9oz) chestnut mushrooms, sliced
2 garlic cloves, crushed
2 × 400g (14oz) cans of chopped tomatoes
1 tablespoon Worcestershire sauce
1 tablespoon tomato purée
1 teaspoon chilli flakes
1 teaspoon dried thyme
250g (9oz) rigatoni
350ml (12fl oz) hot chicken stock
salt and pepper

TO SERVE
chopped parsley leaves
Parmesan cheese, grated (optional)

1. In a large, deep pan (with a lid), fry the chorizo and onions over a medium heat for 10 minutes, stirring occasionally until the onions are soft. Add the mushrooms and garlic and stir them through.
2. Pour in the chopped tomatoes and add the Worcestershire sauce, tomato purée, chilli flakes and thyme.
3. Stir in the rigatoni, then pour in the hot stock. Season with salt and pepper, then place the lid on the pan and allow to gently bubble away for 30 minutes, stirring a couple of times while it's cooking to prevent sticking.
4. Remove the lid from the pan and check the pasta is fully cooked (if not, place the lid back on and cook for 5 more minutes before checking again). If the sauce is looking a little watery, just bubble it over a high heat with the lid off for a few minutes to thicken it up.
5. Serve with parsley scattered over the top, and some Parmesan, if you like.

NOTE You can use any shape of pasta you like for this, but the cooking time may vary. If you want to add extra vegetables, some cherry tomatoes, roasted red pepper, courgette and celery all work well. To make this vegetarian, omit the chorizo and use spray oil to cook the onions in step 1, adding some extra vegetables and 1 teaspoon of smoked paprika. In step 4, swap the chicken stock for vegetable stock, and use Parmesan-style vegetarian cheese to serve

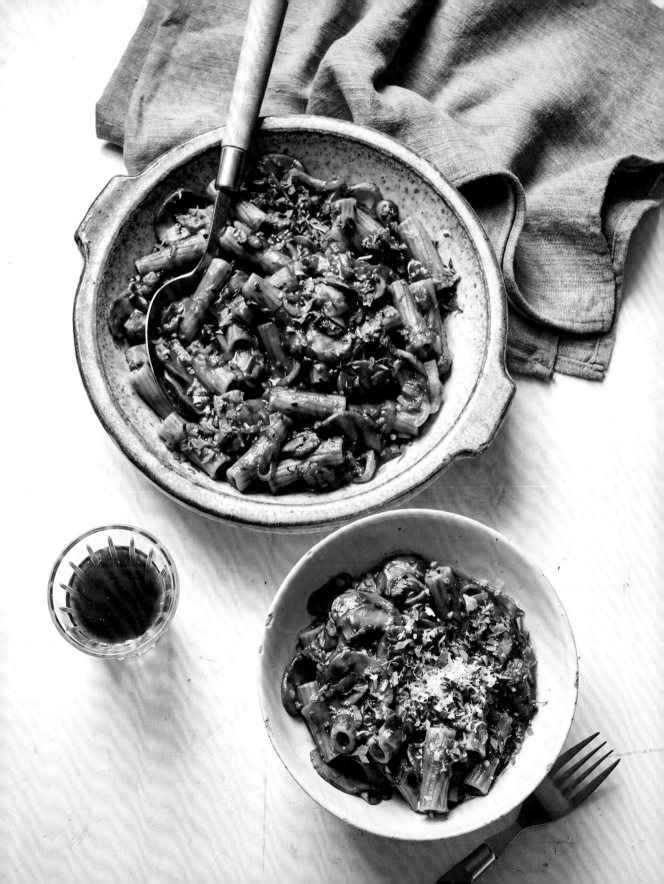

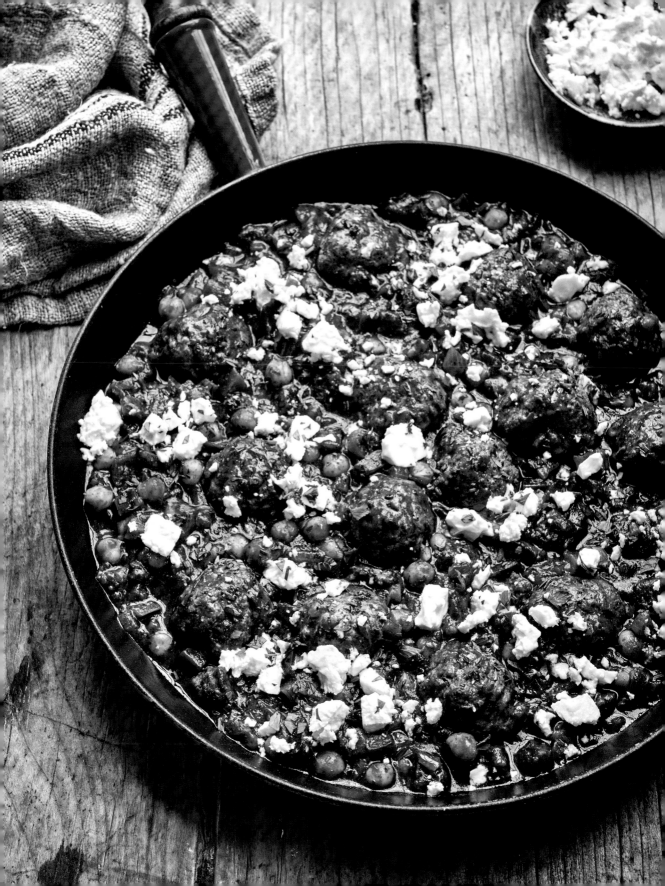

KOFTA MEATBALLS
WITH HARISSA CHICKPEA SAUCE

Harissa, a North African chilli paste, is usually made from red pepper and chilli with a sweet and smoky flavour. You can pick up a jar from most supermarkets, in the section with the herbs and spices. I like to serve this dish with homemade Wholemeal Pitta Bread (see page 202).

CALORIES PER SERVING: 375
PREP TIME: 15 MINUTES
COOK TIME: 35 MINUTES

500g (1lb 2oz) minced lamb (the leanest you can find)
1 teaspoon dried mint
1 teaspoon sumac
½ teaspoon ground cumin
½ teaspoon ground coriander
½ teaspoon garlic granules
½ teaspoon onion granules
1 small egg, lightly beaten
spray oil
1 onion, finely chopped
1 aubergine, finely chopped
2 garlic cloves, crushed
400g (14oz) can of chopped tomatoes
2 tablespoons harissa paste
350ml (12fl oz) hot chicken stock
1 tablespoon dried oregano
400g (14oz) can of chickpeas, drained and rinsed
2 tablespoons tomato purée
juice of 1 lemon
salt and pepper

TO SERVE
mint or parsley leaves, chopped
crumbled feta cheese (optional)

1. Make up the meatballs. In a large bowl, mix the minced lamb, dried mint, sumac, cumin, coriander, garlic granules, onion granules and the egg to combine. Season the mix with salt and pepper.
2. Roll the mixture into mini meatballs, about 2.5cm (1 inch) in diameter.
3. Spray a sauté pan with oil and fry the meatballs over a high heat for 2 minutes, then add the onion, aubergine and garlic and fry for 6 minutes over a medium heat, stirring occasionally.
4. Pour in the chopped tomatoes, then stir in the harissa paste, hot stock, oregano, chickpeas, tomato purée and lemon juice. Season with salt and pepper and allow to simmer gently for 25 minutes.
5. Serve with chopped mint or parsley, adding crumbled feta cheese, if you like.

HOW TO USE LEFTOVER HARISSA:
- Mix it into roasted vegetables.
- Use it as a rub on chicken or salmon before grilling, or on a leg of lamb before roasting.
- Mix it into couscous along with some finely chopped preserved lemons.
- Add some lemon juice and use it as a salad dressing.
- Whisk it into yogurt as a cold sauce to go alongside meat or drizzled over roasted vegetables.
- Add it to a tomato-based pasta sauce.

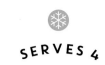

SAUCY SPAG BOL

I am the queen of spaghetti Bolognese! It's always been one of my favourite meals and I'm constantly striving for the perfect recipe. Bolognese itself might not be new, but this method to cook it all in one pan is a bit of a game-changer when you are looking for convenience and speed. Usually I recommend cooking Bolognese sauce for at least 40 minutes to develop the flavours and break down the tomatoes, but this is ready in 25 minutes and still tastes great. This extra-saucy version goes down really well with my kids, I chop the vegetables up extra-small so they don't pick them out and they like the smooth passata in the sauce.

CALORIES PER SERVING: 469
PREP TIME: 10 MINUTES
COOK TIME: 25 MINUTES

spray oil
1 onion, very finely chopped
500g (1lb 2oz) lean minced beef
    (less than 5 per cent fat)
3 garlic cloves, crushed
1 large carrot, peeled and very
    finely chopped
1 tablespoon dark soy sauce
1 tablespoon Italian seasoning
500ml (18fl oz) tomato passata
500ml (18fl oz) hot beef stock
250g (9oz) spaghetti, broken
    in half
salt and pepper

TO SERVE
parsley or basil leaves
Parmesan cheese, grated

1. Spray a sauté pan (with a lid) with oil, then fry the onion, minced beef, garlic and carrot for 8 minutes, stirring and breaking up any clumps in the meat (I use a wooden spoon for this).
2. Stir in salt and pepper, the soy sauce and Italian seasoning. Pour in the passata and hot stock and bring to the boil.
3. Add the broken spaghetti to the sauce, make sure it's all submerged and simmer fast for 15 minutes. Give it the occasional stir with a wooden spoon and try and shuffle the pasta to prevent it from sticking together (make sure it stays submerged though). Place the lid on for the final 5 minutes of cooking.
4. Stir well and test that the spaghetti is cooked through. If it isn't quite cooked and the pan is a little dry, add a splash of boiling water, pop the lid on and cook for a few more minutes before checking again.
5. Serve scattered with herbs and a little Parmesan.

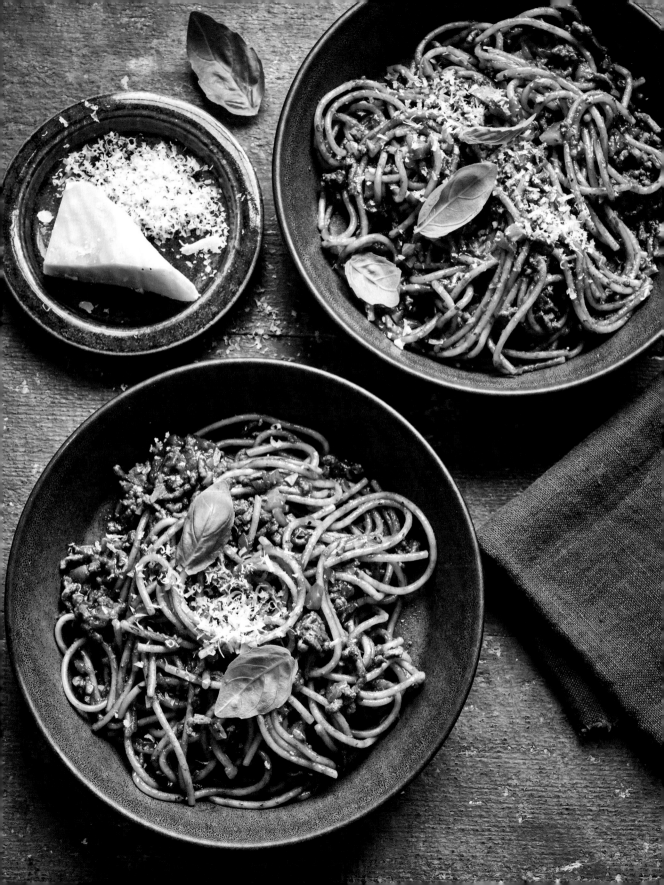

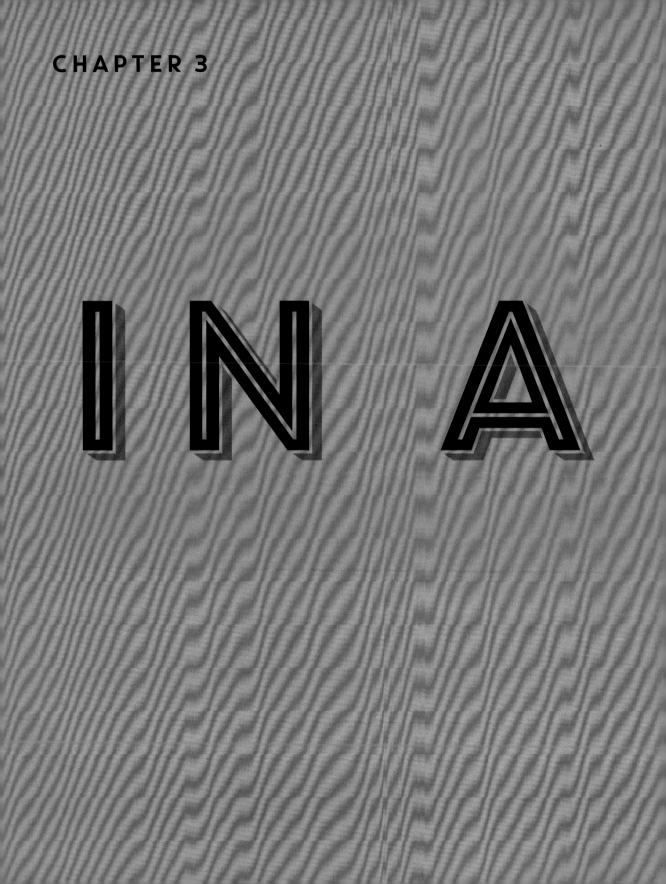

CHAPTER 3

IN A

TRAY

HARISSA BAKED EGGS IN MUSHROOM CUPS
WITH TOMATOES & ASPARAGUS

A very simple but tasty brunch. There is something so satisfying about an egg baking neatly in the cup of a big mushroom (make sure that you select mushrooms with nice deep caps and not flat ones, as you want the egg to neatly sit inside). I like this with toast, or salad leaves.

CALORIES PER SERVING: 134
PREP TIME: 5 MINUTES
COOK TIME: 25 MINUTES

2 portobello mushrooms, stalks removed (see recipe introduction)
150g (5½oz) cherry tomatoes on the vine
spray oil
1 teaspoon harissa paste, or other chilli sauce
2 small eggs
125g (4½oz) fine asparagus spears, woody ends trimmed away
salt and pepper
parsley leaves, chopped, to serve

1. Preheat the oven to 240°C/220°C fan (475°F), Gas Mark 9.
2. Place the mushrooms cap-side down on a baking tray and arrange the tomatoes around them. Spray the mushrooms and tomatoes with a little oil and pop into the oven to bake for 18 minutes.
3. Remove the tray from the oven. Turn the mushrooms over so they are cap-side up. Spoon ½ teaspoon of harissa into each mushroom cap and spread it around.
4. Crack an egg into a small bowl and tip carefully into a mushroom cap. Repeat with the other egg and mushroom cap. Try to keep them contained in the mushrooms, but if they overspill slightly it's not the end of the world!
5. Arrange the asparagus in any gaps around the tray and spray with a little more oil, then season everything with salt and pepper.
6. Carefully return the tray to the oven, trying not to spill the egg. Bake for 4 minutes, in which time the white of the egg should be cooked through but the yolk should still be runny. Serve immediately, scattered with parsley.

NOTE You can tailor these, or beef up the meal to your own taste. Add some baby spinach to the tray at the same time as the asparagus in step 5, or add bacon to the tray when you first roast the tomatoes and mushrooms in step 2.

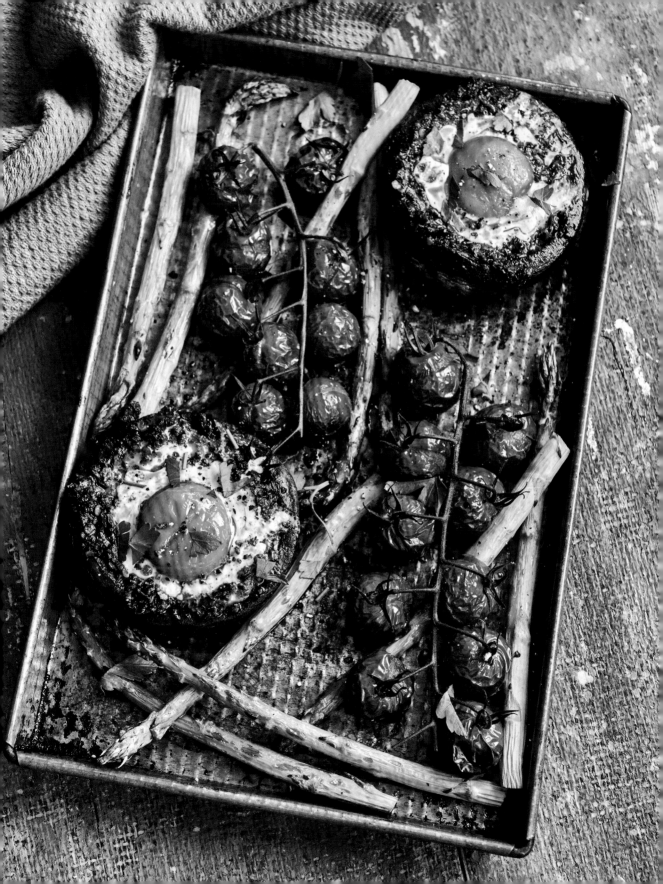

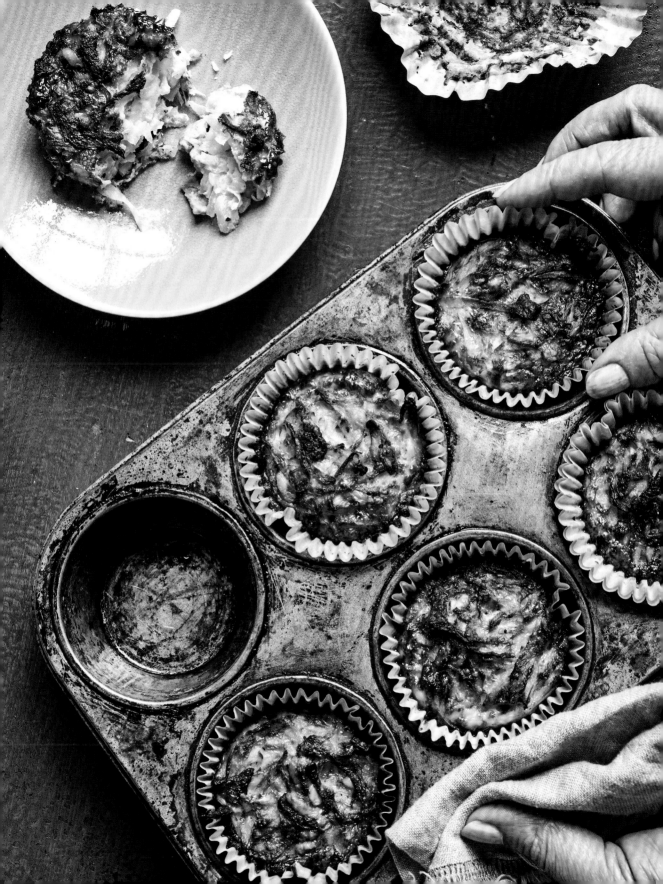

RÖSTI BREAKFAST MUFFINS

These make a great all-in-one breakfast. Delicious fresh from the oven, or they can also be reheated another day if you have leftovers. I love wrapping these up in foil while they are still warm and taking them for a breakfast picnic on the beach.

CALORIES PER MUFFIN: 123
PREP TIME: 15 MINUTES
COOK TIME: 25 MINUTES

400g (14oz) potatoes, peeled
  and grated
1 red onion, grated
2 smoked bacon medallions,
  finely chopped
30g (1oz) mature Cheddar
  cheese, grated
2 large eggs
½ teaspoon salt
pepper
low-calorie cooking spray

1. Preheat the oven to 240°C/220°C fan (475°F), Gas Mark 9.
2. Squeeze the water out from the grated potatoes. I put them into a colander and hold it over the sink, pressing down firmly on the potatoes to squeeze the water out. You can also do it with a salad spinner.
3. In a large bowl, mix all the ingredients together except the low-calorie cooking spray.
4. Place 6 muffin cases into a muffin tray and spray them with low-calorie cooking spray.
5. Divide the mixture evenly between the cases, spray the tops with low-calorie cooking spray and bake in the oven for 25 minutes. The tops should be golden brown with crispy bits.

NOTE Some extra ingredients that you could add are chopped roast peppers, spring onions, chives, spinach, grated sweet potato and chilli. You can also swap the bacon for chorizo, or experiment with some different cheeses, such as feta and Gruyère.

ASPARAGUS & GRUYÈRE QUICHE
WITH SWEET POTATO CRUST

Sweet potato makes a fantastic alternative to pastry in a quiche.
It's not as dense as pastry, and as it shrinks when baking there will be
gaps along the way (so don't make the mistake of using a loose-based
quiche tin or you will have leakage!) but it still forms an outer crust
that gives structure and adds a really lovely sweet flavour.

CALORIES PER SERVING: 261
PREP TIME: 10 MINUTES
COOK TIME: 35 MINUTES

low-calorie cooking spray
4 medium sweet potatoes (total
   weight 250–300g/9–10½oz),
   peeled and finely sliced
6 large eggs
60g (2¼oz) Gruyère cheese,
   grated
8 asparagus spears, woody ends
   trimmed away, sliced on the
   diagonal into 2cm (¾ inch)
   pieces
salt and pepper

1. Preheat the oven to 220°C/200°C fan (425°F), Gas Mark 7.
2. Spray a solid-based 22cm (8½ inch) quiche dish with low-calorie cooking spray and layer the sweet potato slices from the middle to the outside, overlapping them and working in a circular motion until the base is covered. Lay the rest of the potato slices around the edge of the dish, again overlapping them (halve them if you need to make them fit), then spray with low-calorie cooking spray. Place in the oven and bake for 15 minutes.
3. Meanwhile, prepare the filling. In a large bowl, beat the eggs, season with salt and pepper and add half the grated cheese. Mix in the asparagus.
4. Remove the baked quiche crust from the oven and reduce the oven temperature to 200°C/180°C fan (400°F), Gas Mark 6. Pour the egg mixture into the sweet potato crust and sprinkle the remaining cheese over to evenly cover.
5. Bake for 20 minutes, it will be browned (but not burned) on top and some of the exposed sweet potato pieces will have charred edges.
6. Slice into 4 and use a pie slice to carefully remove from the dish. Serve warm or cold.

NOTE Try swapping the Gruyère and asparagus for roasted peppers, spring onions, jalapeños, smoked paprika and red Leicester cheese, added with the egg in step 3.

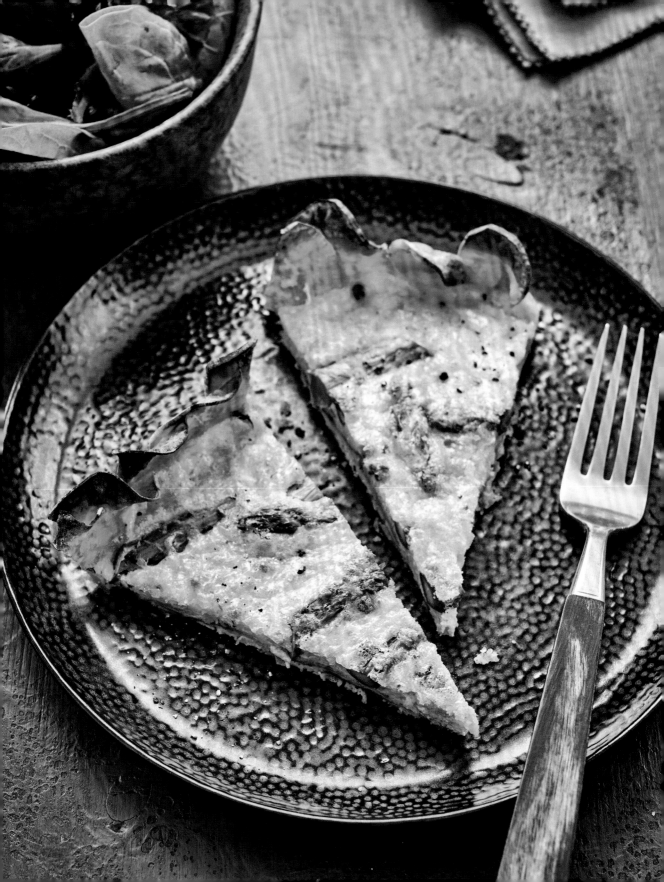

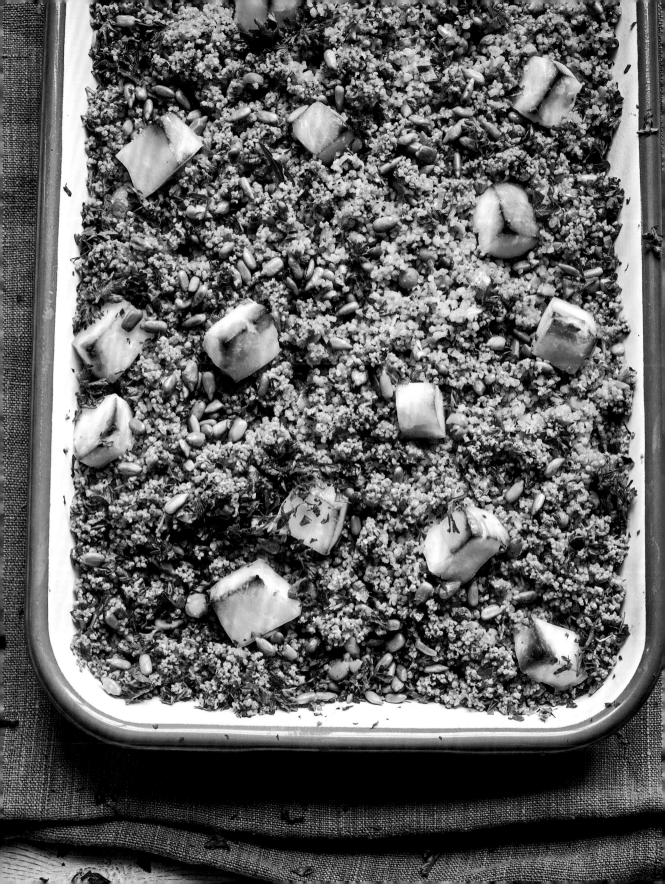

ZINGY COUSCOUS
WITH HALLOUMI CUBES

This full-of-flavour green-hued couscous is flavoured with pops of zingy preserved lemon and topped with little salty squares of baked halloumi. You can find an easy-peasy recipe for making your own Speedy Preserved Lemons in this book (see page 209), or you can buy them in larger supermarkets. Preserved lemons are a magic ingredient for adding bags of flavour to grains such as couscous, bulgur wheat and quinoa.

CALORIES PER SERVING: 470
PREP TIME: 15 MINUTES,
PLUS SOAKING TIME
COOK TIME: 20 MINUTES

300g (10½oz) wholewheat couscous

500ml (18fl oz) hot vegetable stock

200g (7oz) frozen peas, defrosted

handful of baby spinach

small handful of mint leaves

1 garlic clove

6 spring onions, sliced

2 slices (total weight 30g/1oz) preserved lemons, finely chopped, any pips removed

1 red chilli, deseeded and finely chopped

140g (5oz) halloumi cheese, chopped into small cubes

2 tablespoons sunflower seeds

salt and pepper

chopped parsley leaves, to serve

1. Preheat the oven to 180°C/160°C fan (350°F), Gas Mark 4.

2. Pour the couscous into a medium-sized heatproof bowl and pour in 350ml (12fl oz) of the hot stock. Cover with a plate or foil and leave for 10 minutes.

3. Meanwhile, use a mini chopper to blend together the peas, spinach, mint, garlic and 3 of the spring onions with the remaining 150ml (¼ pint) of stock. Add the purée to the couscous, season with salt and pepper and stir in the preserved lemons and chilli.

4. Spread out the couscous in a small baking tray or dish (I used a rectangular dish, 24 × 19cm/9½ × 7½ inches). Scatter the halloumi and sunflower seeds over, then bake in the oven for 20 minutes. The halloumi should be browning on the edges, and the sunflower seeds lightly toasted. Scatter with parsley to serve.

NOTE If you want to add extra green vegetables to this, just slice them up and stir them in before spreading out the couscous on the tray in step 4. You could use asparagus, broccoli, green beans or courgette. Chopped roast red peppers also work well.

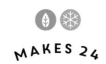

SPICED SNACK BITES

Great little snack-sized bites similar to pakoras to go alongside a curry, salad, or simply to be eaten as a healthy snack. They are delicious warm or cold. Chickpeas form the base, with mild curry flavours and cauliflower, sweet carrot and peas.

CALORIES PER SNACK BITE: 26
PREP TIME: 15 MINUTES
COOK TIME: 35 MINUTES

400g (14oz) can of chickpeas, drained and rinsed

1 garlic clove

1 small egg

3 small carrots (total weight about 180g/6¼oz), peeled and roughly chopped

2 spring onions, roughly chopped

1 tablespoon mild curry powder

½ teaspoon salt, plus extra to serve

100g (3½oz) frozen peas, defrosted

½ cauliflower, roughly chopped

low-calorie cooking spray

1. Preheat the oven to 220°C/200°C fan (425°F), Gas Mark 7.
2. Using a food processor, blend the chickpeas, garlic, egg, carrots, spring onions, curry powder and salt until you have a rough paste. Add the peas and cauliflower and blend until both are roughly chopped and blended.
3. Line a large baking tray (or 2 smaller ones) with baking parchment and spray with low-calorie cooking spray. Form the mixture into 24 small patties with your hands, laying out on the tray as you go.
4. Spray the patties with low-calorie cooking spray, then bake on the middle shelf of the oven for 35 minutes. The snack bites should be golden brown and crisp on the outside and soft in the middle. Sprinkle with salt and serve hot.

NOTE Customize these with your favourite vegetables, such as spinach, red peppers or green beans. If you like things extra-spicy, then add some chilli or chilli powder.

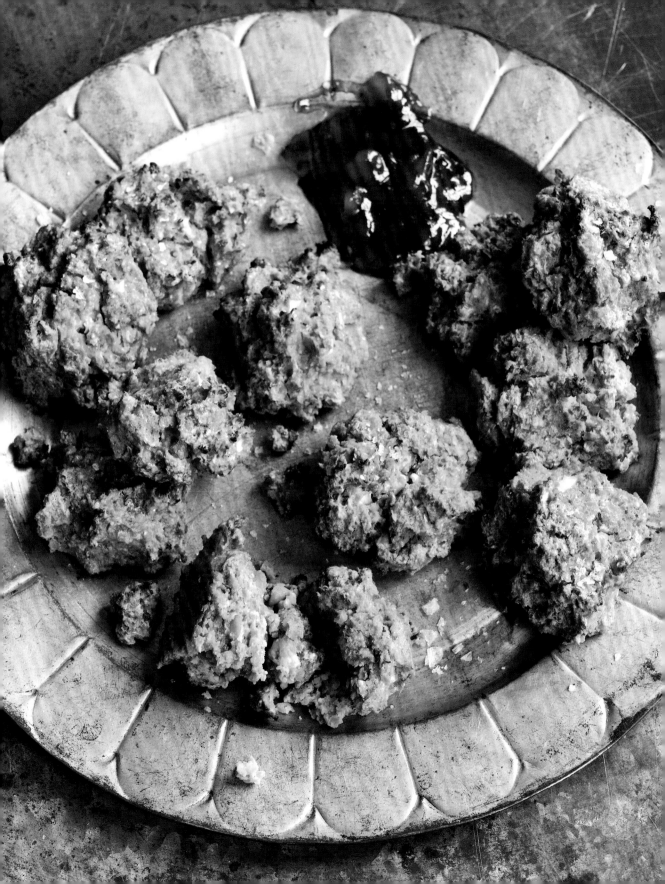

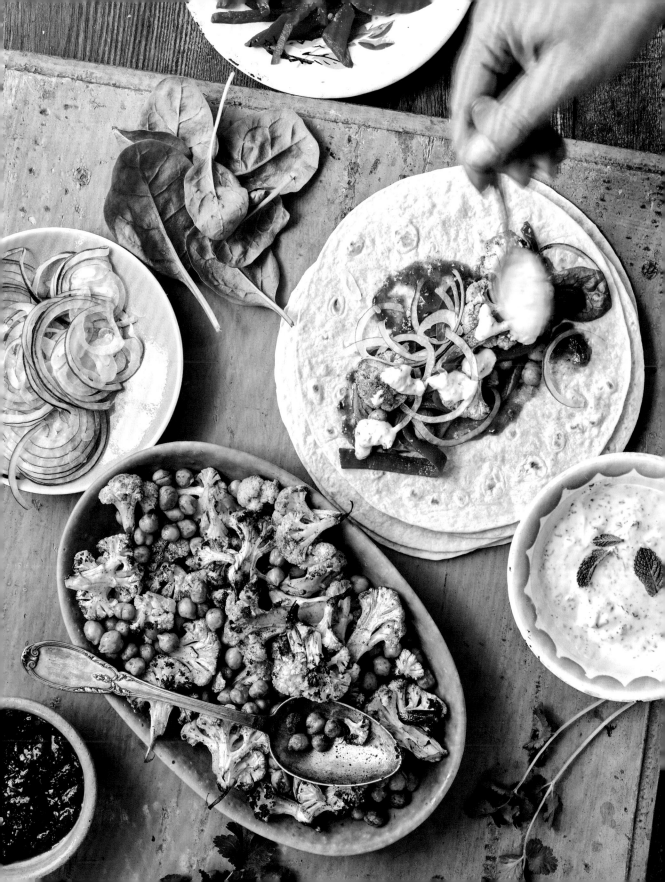

BOMBAY BURRITOS

These burritos make a great lunch, either warm or cold. Roasted, spiced chickpeas and cauliflower make up the hearty filling, with spinach, mango chutney and a cool mint yogurt supplying the high notes. Great with some Quick Purple Pickle (see page 210) too.

CALORIES PER SERVING: 300
PREP TIME: 20 MINUTES
COOK TIME: 25 MINUTES

1 cauliflower, cut into florets
low-calorie cooking spray
400g (14oz) can of chickpeas, drained and rinsed
1 tablespoon Tandoori-style Spice Blend (for homemade see page 222)
6 medium-sized low-fat tortilla wraps
6 teaspoons mango chutney
50g (1¾oz) baby spinach
2 roasted red peppers in brine (total weight about 160g/5¾oz), drained and finely sliced
½ red onion, very finely sliced
coriander leaves
chilli sauce (optional)
salt and pepper

MINTED YOGURT

8 tablespoons fat-free Greek yogurt
small handful of mint leaves
1 garlic clove
juice of ½ lemon
½ teaspoon coarse sea salt

1. Preheat the oven to 240°C/220°C fan (475°F), Gas Mark 9.

2. Make up the minted yogurt by using a mini chopper to blend the yogurt, mint leaves, garlic, lemon juice and salt into a smooth dressing, then set aside.

3. Cover a baking tray with baking parchment, spread the cauliflower over it in an even layer and spray with low-calorie cooking spray. Roast for 10 minutes, then remove from the oven, mix the cauliflower around, add the chickpeas, Tandoori-style spice blend and salt and pepper, spray with more low-calorie cooking spray and roast for another 15 minutes. Remove from the oven.

4. Assemble the burritos. Warm the tortillas in the microwave according to the package instructions. Lay each tortilla out and spread 1 teaspoon of mango chutney around the centre. Add a small handful of the baby spinach, then some cauliflower and chickpeas. Add some roast red pepper, a few slivers of red onion, then dress with minted yogurt. Scatter over coriander and add chilli sauce, if you wish.

5. Roll up into burritos (see below) and serve.

> **HOW TO ROLL A BURRITO**
> Warming the wraps before folding ensures they are pliable. Put the fillings in the centre and towards the top of the wrap. Fold the bottom up over the fillings, then fold in the two sides. I keep the top open so the fillings come just to the edge (if you are using larger tortillas you can close the top end too). Hold the folds firmly in place, then wrap the burritos in foil to keep them together.

BAKED PRAWN, LEMON & CHILLI RISOTTO

An irresistible combination of flavours in the easiest risotto you will ever make! Risotto rice (carnaroli or arborio) actually holds up really well to oven baking, as it has a firm texture which – as long as it's not overcooked – will not turn mushy.

CALORIES PER SERVING: 353
PREP TIME: 10 MINUTES
COOK TIME: 50 MINUTES

low-calorie cooking spray
250g (9oz) cherry tomatoes
1 red onion, finely chopped
2 garlic cloves, finely chopped
1 unwaxed lemon, zested, then
   cut into wedges
150g (5½oz) cooked and peeled
   king prawns
300g (10½oz) risotto rice
   (carnaroli or arborio)
1 litre (1¾ pints) hot chicken
   stock
150g (5½oz) fine asparagus
   spears, woody ends trimmed
   away
salt and pepper
parsley leaves, finely chopped,
   to serve

1. Preheat the oven to 220°C/200°C fan (425°F), Gas Mark 7.
2. Spray an oven dish (I use a rectangular dish 24 × 19cm/ 9½ × 7½ inches) with low-calorie cooking spray and add the tomatoes, onion and garlic. Mix and spray again with low-calorie cooking spray. Place into the oven and cook for 20 minutes.
3. Remove the dish from the oven, stir in the lemon zest and prawns, season with salt and pepper, then stir in the rice. Pour the hot stock over, then carefully return the dish to the oven. Bake for 25 minutes
4. Remove the dish from the oven, use a fork to stir and mix the risotto, then place the asparagus on top, season with salt and pepper and spray with low-calorie cooking spray. Return to the oven to cook for a final 5 minutes.
5. Serve with lemon wedges and finely chopped parsley.

NOTE Make this vegetarian by replacing the prawns with 2 roasted and chopped red peppers and substituting the chicken stock for vegetable stock.

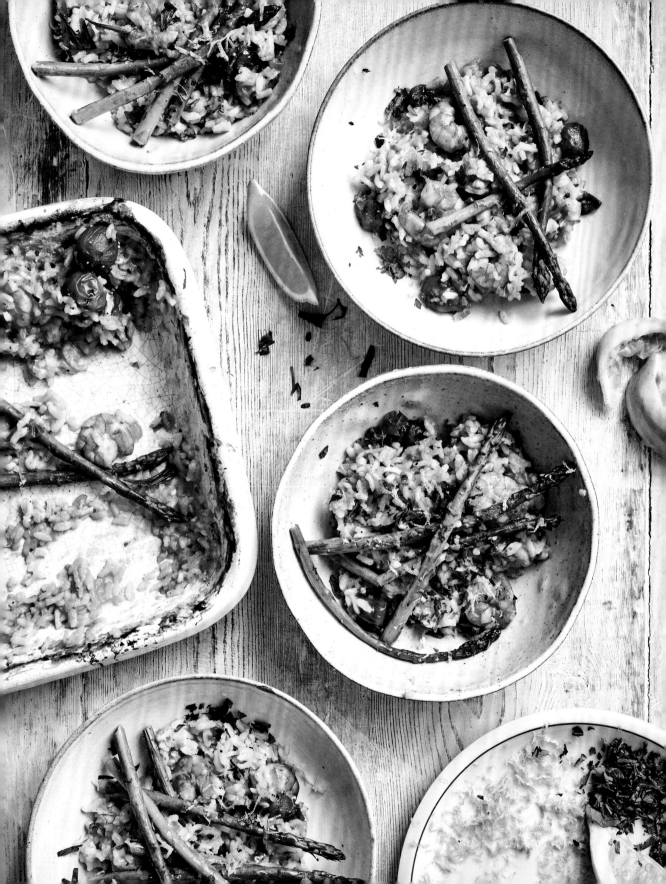

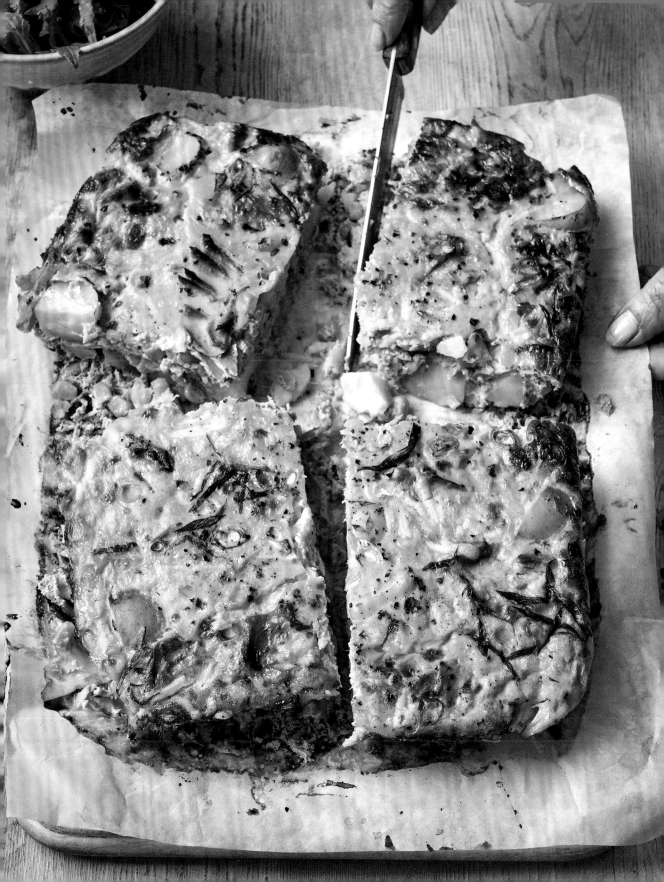

TUNA & SWEETCORN BAKED FRITTATA

Oven-baked frittatas are one of the easiest meals to have up your sleeve. They require little work, you can use up so many different ingredients and they are delicious hot and cold. This frittata uses the classic mix of tuna and sweetcorn to make a filling dish that is family friendly, and ideal for a meal, snack or picnic. Canned new potatoes might sound like an odd ingredient, but they are great in this, saving you the job of pre-cooking potatoes and meaning that the recipe is made from ingredients that you can have handy in the cupboard.

CALORIES PER SERVING: 321
PREP TIME: 5 MINUTES
COOK TIME: 25 MINUTES

6 large eggs
125ml (4fl oz) semi-skimmed milk
2 × 145g (5¼oz) cans of tuna in spring water, drained
40g (1½oz) Cheddar cheese, grated
2 teaspoons finely chopped tarragon, plus tarragon sprigs to serve
low-calorie cooking spray
540g (1lb 3½oz) canned new potatoes in water, drained and chopped into bite-sized pieces
2 spring onions, finely sliced
200g (7oz) can of sweetcorn, drained
salt and pepper

1. Preheat the oven to 200°C/180°C fan (400°F), Gas Mark 6.
2. In a large bowl, beat the eggs, then add the milk and tuna, half the Cheddar, the tarragon and some salt and pepper. Mix well.
3. Line a baking dish or tray (measuring about 25 × 21cm/ 10 × 8¼ inches) with baking paper and spray with low-calorie cooking spray.
4. Spread the potatoes out into the dish and scatter over the spring onions and sweetcorn. Pour over the egg mix and sprinkle over the remaining Cheddar.
5. Bake on the middle shelf of the oven for 25 minutes. The top should be golden brown and set through. Serve with a few fresh tarragon leaves scattered over the top.

NOTE Tarragon has a distinct aniseed flavour, which tastes gorgeous in this, but if you are making this for children you may wish to replace it with something with a milder flavour, such as parsley, or leave it out entirely. Other ingredients which you could add to this frittata are spinach, kale, asparagus and cherry tomatoes.

SWEET CHILLI SALMON MUDDLE

This is a simple, healthy midweek meal that you can throw together in no time. Sweet chilli sauce is a really versatile ingredient to have in the cupboard, to add a quick burst of flavour to meals. I like this with mixed salad leaves on the side.

CALORIES PER SERVING: 449
PREP TIME: 10 MINUTES
COOK TIME: 45 MINUTES

4 tablespoons sweet chilli sauce
2 tablespoons light soy sauce
juice of 1 lime, plus lime wedges
  to serve
700g (1lb 9oz) sweet potatoes,
  peeled and cut into bite-sized
  chunks
2 red onions, cut into wedges
1 red pepper, deseeded and
  chopped
1 yellow pepper, deseeded and
  chopped
1 teaspoon olive oil
4 salmon fillets
coriander leaves, to serve

1. Preheat the oven to 220°C/200°C fan (425°F), Gas Mark 7.
2. Make up a sauce in a small bowl by mixing together the sweet chilli sauce, soy sauce and lime juice.
3. Prepare the vegetables and place into a large bowl. Stir in the olive oil to coat, then stir in half the sauce.
4. In a large baking tray (mine measured 34 × 24cm/ 13½ × 9½ inches), spread out the vegetables and roast for 30 minutes, giving them a stir halfway though. After 30 minutes, give the vegetables another stir, then place the salmon fillets on top. Spoon the remaining sauce over the fish.
5. Return the tray to the oven and roast for 15 minutes. After this time the salmon should be perfectly cooked and the vegetables roasted with some slightly blackened edges. Serve immediately scattered with coriander and with lime wedges on the side.

NOTE If you wish to add some extra green vegetables such as green beans, broccoli or asparagus, add them with the salmon in step 4 and give them a little spray with oil or low-calorie cooking spray.

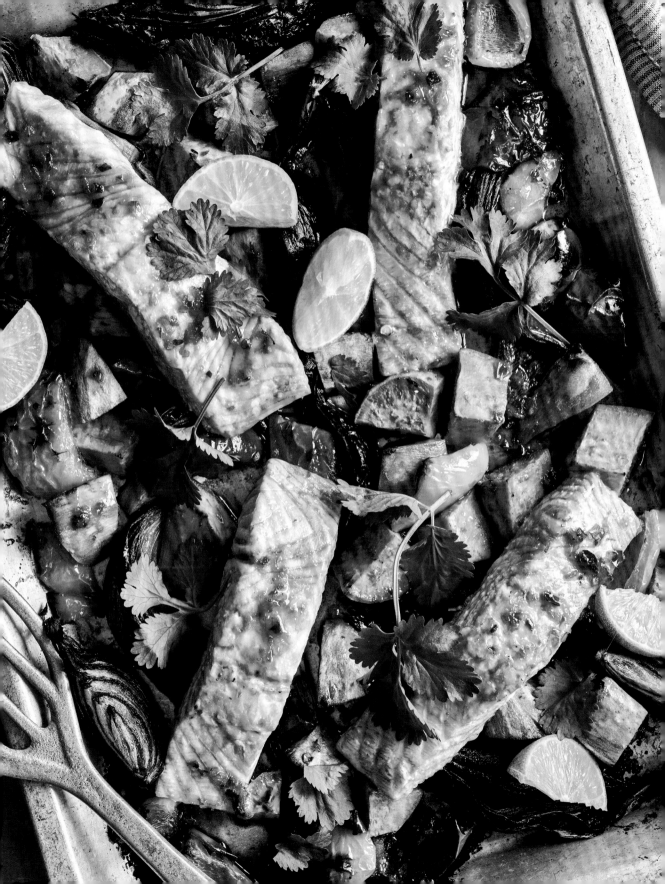

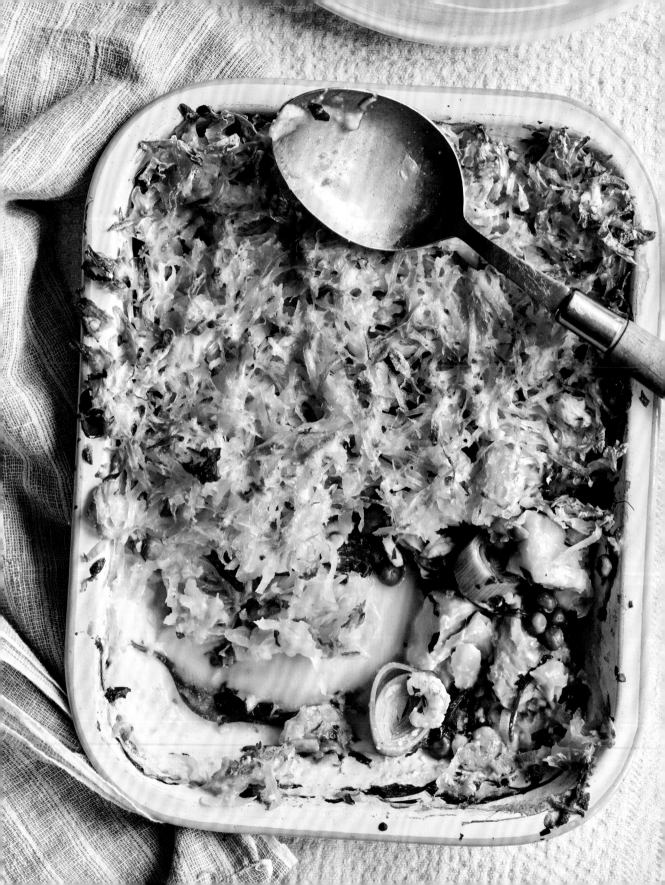

RÖSTI-TOPPED FISH PIE

A rösti topping is a great way to make a fish pie without having to boil and mash potatoes and it adds a lovely crispness to the topping. If you can get hold of samphire (you can find it in larger supermarkets and at fishmongers), it makes a great side dish.

CALORIES PER SERVING: 512
PREP TIME: 20 MINUTES
COOK TIME: 40 MINUTES

250–300g (9–10½oz) skinless firm white fish fillets, such as basa, cod or haddock, chopped into chunks

1 smoked mackerel fillet (about 80g/2¾oz), skinned and chopped

80g (2¾oz) small cooked and peeled cold-water prawns

1 leek, trimmed and finely sliced

3 tablespoons cornflour

300ml (½ pint) semi-skimmed milk

80g (2¾oz) garlic and herb roulé soft cheese

finely grated zest of 1 unwaxed lemon

100g (3½oz) baby spinach, roughly chopped

large handful of parsley leaves, chopped

100g (3½oz) frozen peas, defrosted

60g (2½oz) mature Cheddar cheese, grated

700g (1lb 9oz) potatoes, peeled

spray oil, or low-calorie cooking spray

salt and pepper

1. Preheat the oven to 200°C/180°C fan (400°F), Gas Mark 6.
2. Put the white fish in a large bowl with the mackerel, prawns and leek and stir in 2 tablespoons of the cornflour to coat.
3. In a small jug, measure out the milk and mix in the garlic and herb cheese with a fork: it should melt into the milk and thicken it up, but it doesn't matter if there are a few lumps. Pour this mixture in with the fish. Add the lemon zest, baby spinach, parsley, peas and half the Cheddar, season with salt and pepper, then give it all a thorough mix. In a deep baking dish (mine measured 25 × 22cm/ 10 × 8½ inches), spread the fish mixture out evenly.
4. Grate the potatoes into a colander, hold it over the sink and squeeze down to push out as much liquid as possible. If you prefer, you can place these in a clean muslin to squeeze out the liquid. (If you are grating the potatoes in advance, cover in cold water until ready to use, so they don't go brown, then drain and squeeze out excess liquid when you are ready).
5. Stir the remaining 1 tablespoon of cornflour into the grated potatoes, then stir in the remaining Cheddar. Spread the grated potatoes evenly over the pie, and spray with oil or low-calorie cooking spray.
6. Bake on the middle shelf of the oven for 40 minutes, until the top of the pie is golden brown, with crisp edges.

NOTE You can substitute the white fish for salmon in this. If you want to avoid the smoked flavour that mackerel gives, simply replace it with extra prawns or white fish.

FANCY CHICKEN KIEVS

WITH ROASTED TOMATOES & ASPARAGUS

This has always been one of the favourite quick and easy dinners in my house. Just a few simple ingredients creates something that is so full of flavour and feels utterly indulgent.

CALORIES PER SERVING: 351
PREP TIME: 5 MINUTES
COOK TIME: 25 MINUTES

2 skinless chicken breasts
40g (1½oz) garlic & herb roulé
   soft cheese
4 slices of prosciutto
spray oil
220g (7¾oz) cherry tomatoes
   on the vine
125g (4½oz) asparagus spears,
   woody ends trimmed away
coarse sea salt

1. Preheat the oven to 210°C/190°C fan (410°F), Gas Mark 6½.
2. Slice the chicken breasts down the middle lengthways, being sure only to slice halfway through. Stuff each breast with half the cheese. Wrap each stuffed breast in 2 slices of prosciutto, paying attention to cover the split which contains the cheese.
3. Spray a baking tray or shallow oven dish with spray oil and place the chicken breasts in. Place the tomatoes (still on the vine) in the dish and spray with a little extra oil.
4. Roast for 15 minutes. Remove the tray from the oven, place the asparagus around the chicken and tomatoes and roast for a further 10 minutes.
5. Check that the chicken is cooked through (slice through the thickest part and check for any sign of pink; roast for a final few minutes if it is not ready before checking again). Place on warmed plates. Grind a little salt over the asparagus and tomatoes and spoon any juice left in the tray around the chicken, then serve.

NOTE Other vegetables you could add to roast in this bake are red onions, field mushrooms, courgettes, peppers and fennel (add these with the chicken in step 3), or green beans, cauliflower and Tenderstem broccoli (add these with the asparagus in step 4).

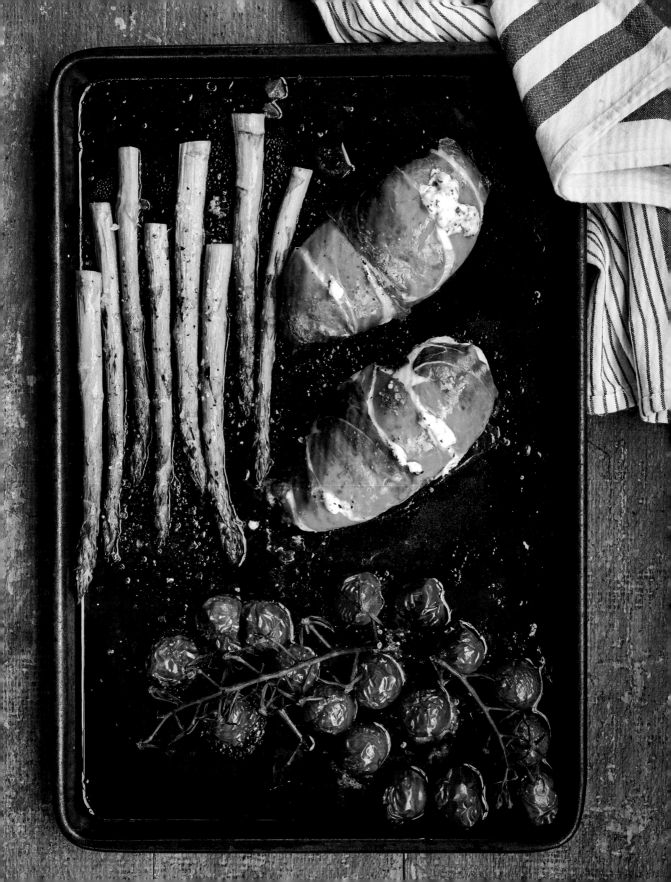

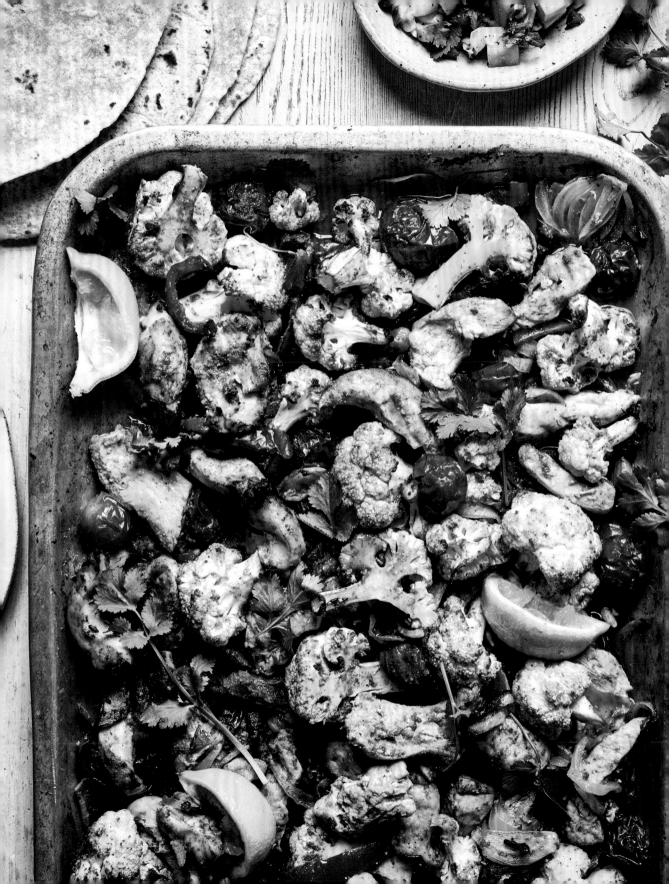

CURRIED CHICKEN BAKE

A classic that always goes down a treat, but an easy version all made in one tray, with no need to pre-fry it or otherwise tend to it. Roasting it in this way allows the peppers and onions to develop deep flavour. The added cauliflower makes it a filling meal-in-one. If you're hungry, serve with mini naans or chapatis on the side.

CALORIES PER SERVING: 272
PREP-TIME: 10 MINUTES
COOK TIME: 40 MINUTES

3 skinless chicken breasts, sliced
   into strips
3 peppers, deseeded and sliced
   into strips
2 onions, sliced
250g (9oz) cherry tomatoes
low-calorie cooking spray
1 cauliflower, broken into florets
3 tablespoons red wine vinegar

FOR THE SPICE MIX
2 teaspoons garam masala
2 teaspoons ground turmeric
2 teaspoons garlic granules
1 teaspoon ground ginger
1 teaspoon salt
1 teaspoon chilli powder

TO SERVE
coriander leaves
lemon wedges

1. Preheat the oven to 200°C/180°C fan (400°F), Gas Mark 6.
2. Mix all the ingredients for the spice mix together in a small bowl.
3. Put the chicken in a large baking tray with the peppers, onions and baby tomatoes and mix everything together. Spray with low-calorie cooking spray and bake on the middle shelf of the oven for 20 minutes.
4. After 20 minutes, remove the tray, give everything a stir, then add the spice mix, cauliflower and vinegar. Stir to coat everything in the spices and return to the oven for 20 minutes.
5. Remove the tray from the oven, there should be a little bit of charring on the peppers and cauliflower. Stir everything around; there might be some liquid in the tray and you can stir this all together with the vegetables and meat before serving with coriander leaves and lemon wedges.

MANGO SALSA
I sometimes make a quick mango salsa to serve alongside this. Just finely chop 1 mango, 1 red pepper and ½ cucumber, slice 3 spring onions and mix together in a bowl with ¼ teaspoon ground cumin, the juice of 1 lime, some grindings of coarse sea salt and a handful of chopped coriander leaves.

LEMON & HERB ROAST CHICKEN DINNER

Ideal for a lazy Sunday dinner, using new potatoes for your roast means no par-boiling or multiple elements to juggle. A full meal cooked in one tray, full of Greek-inspired herb and lemon flavours. Make sure to bring the chicken to room temperature by removing it from the refrigerator 30 minutes before cooking.

CALORIES PER SERVING: 554
PREP TIME: 15 MINUTES,
PLUS RESTING TIME
COOK TIME: 1¼ HOURS

1 chicken (about 1.5kg/3lb 5oz)
1 lemon
1 bulb of garlic
spray oil
1kg (2lb 4oz) new potatoes,
    larger ones halved so they are
    all roughly the same size
750g (1lb 10oz) carrots, peeled
    and cut into chunks a similar
    size to the potatoes
400g (14oz) parsnips, peeled
    and cut into chunks
1 tablespoon Greek-style
    Seasoning (see page 222)

1. Preheat the oven to 220°C/200°C fan (425°F), Gas Mark 7.
2. Put the chicken in a large roasting tray. Squeeze the lemon juice over, then stuff the 2 lemon shells into the chicken's cavity. Cover with foil and place on the middle shelf of the oven to roast for 30 minutes.
3. Meanwhile, use a sharp knife to cut about 1cm (½ inch) from the top of the garlic bulb, give it a little spray of oil and wrap it in foil.
4. After 30 minutes, remove the chicken from the oven, take off the foil (reserve it) and spread the potatoes, carrots and parsnips around the chicken. Sprinkle the Greek-style seasoning over everything and spray all over with spray oil. Place the wrapped garlic in the tray, cut-side up.
5. Roast for a further 45 minutes, stirring the vegetables and basting the chicken halfway through. Remove from the oven and check that the chicken is cooked through (I recommend checking using a meat thermometer – insert the probe into the thickest part of the chicken thigh: properly cooked chicken will measure at least 75°C/167°F). Carefully lift the chicken on to a large plate and cover with the reserved foil. Switch the oven off and pop the tray of veg in there to keep warm.
6. Allow the chicken to rest for 15 minutes (this keeps the juices in and the meat succulent).
7. Carve the chicken and serve with the roasted vegetables. The roasted garlic cloves should pop easily out of the skin and be soft; serve these alongside the vegetables.

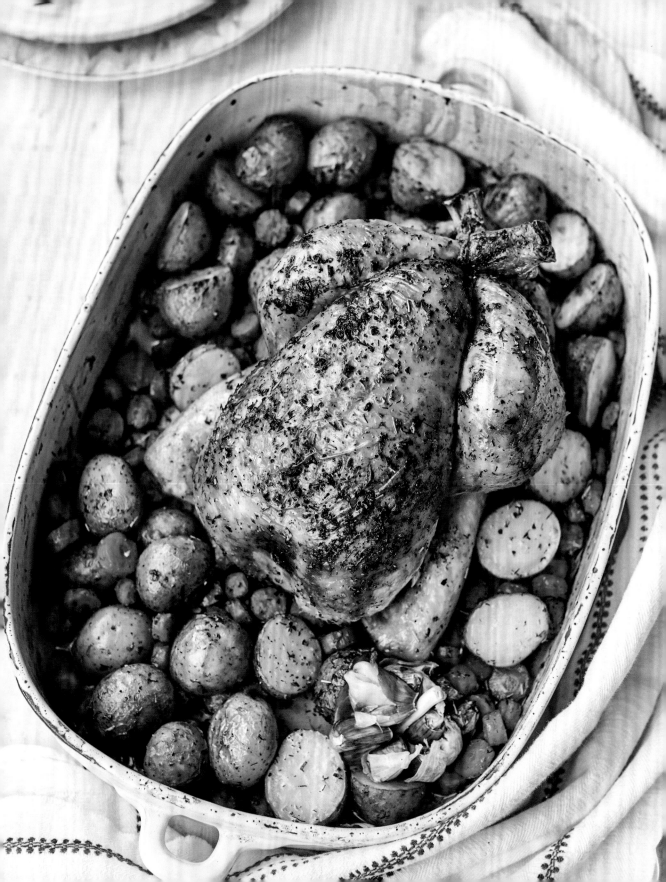

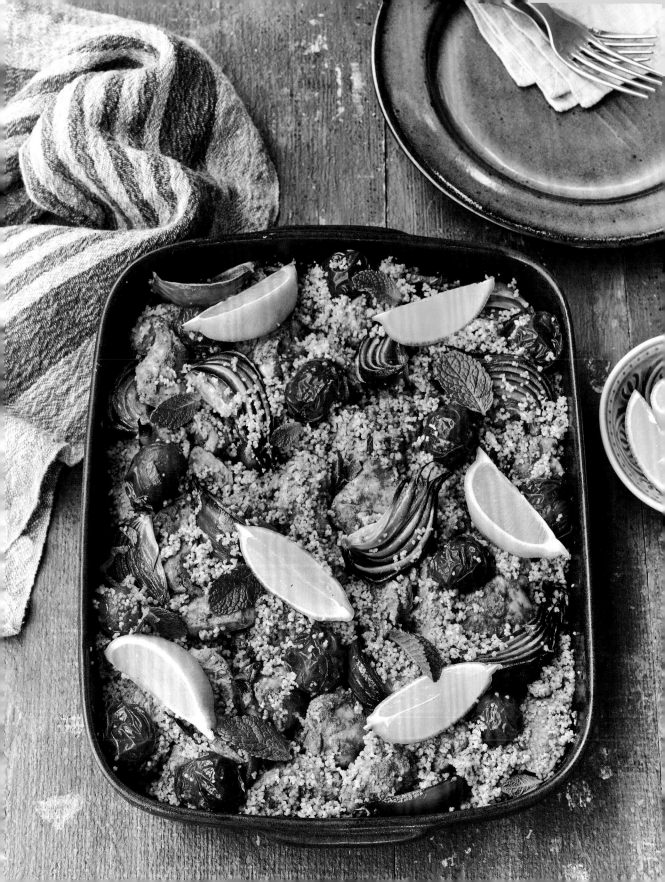

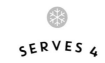

TANDOORI CHICKEN
WITH LEMON & MINT COUSCOUS

Marinating chicken in yogurt and tandoori spices is one of the simplest ways to get amazing flavour into the meat. I use my own homemade Tandoori-style spice blend in this dish, but you can easily pick up a pre-made mix if you don't have time for this step, you may just need to adjust the amount used according to the package instructions.

CALORIES PER SERVING: 411
PREP TIME: 5 MINUTES
COOK TIME: 30 MINUTES

3–4 skinless chicken breasts (total weight about 600g/1lb 5oz), cut into chunks
3 tablespoons Tandoori-style Spice Blend (for homemade, see page 222)
2 garlic cloves, crushed
finely grated zest and juice of 2 unwaxed lemons, plus lemon wedges to serve
3 tablespoons fat-free Greek yogurt
2 red onions, cut into wedges
250ml (9fl oz) hot chicken stock
200g (7oz) baby tomatoes
spray oil
200g (7oz) wholewheat couscous
small handful of mint leaves, finely chopped, plus extra to serve
salt and pepper

1. Preheat the oven to 220°C/200°C fan (425°F), Gas Mark 7.
2. In a bowl, mix the chicken with the tandoori spice blend, garlic, lemon juice and Greek yogurt. Set aside while you prepare the onions and make up the chicken stock.
3. Choose a roasting tin, or shallow ovenproof dish (mine measured 31 × 20cm/12½ × 8 inches). Spread the chicken over the dish, scatter in the tomatoes and onion wedges, spray with spray oil and roast for 25 minutes on the middle shelf of the oven.
4. Measure the couscous into a bowl and stir in the lemon zest and mint. Season with salt and pepper.
5. Remove the tin or dish of chicken from the oven, stir in the couscous and pour over the stock (try to cover all the couscous and ensure the stock reaches the corners of the baking dish). Give another little stir to make sure there are no big dry clumps of couscous, then cover the tin or dish tightly with foil and pop back into the oven to bake for a final 5 minutes.
6. Remove the dish from the oven and take off the foil, use a fork to rake through the couscous and loosen everything up, scatter with mint leaves and serve with lemon wedges.

NOTE If you want extra green vegetables with this, add them on top of the couscous and stock before covering with foil in step 5. Vegetables such as green beans, asparagus and sugarsnap peas will all steam nicely, retaining a fresh bite.

LEMON & GARLIC PORK
WITH HOT POTATO & BEETROOT SALAD

Simple flavours and vibrant colours make this a real summer favourite for me. A mix of potatoes and beetroot makes a great fibre-rich base. Pork tenderloin is an affordable and quick-to-cook cut, ideal for weeknight dinners. You can pick up vacuum-packed cooked beetroot in most supermarkets. Just remember to wear some gloves when preparing it if you don't want purple fingers! I serve this over a small bag of pea shoots or other sweet baby-leaf salad.

CALORIES PER SERVING: 302
PREP TIME: 15 MINUTES, PLUS
RESTING TIME
COOK TIME: 40 MINUTES

500g (1lb 2oz) new potatoes, quartered
spray oil
finely grated zest of 1 unwaxed lemon
1 tablespoon fat-free Greek yogurt
2 garlic cloves, crushed
1 pork tenderloin/fillet (total weight 400–500g/14oz–1lb 2oz)
pinch of sweet paprika
300g (10½oz) cooked beetroot, cut into 2cm (¾ inch) chunks
1 teaspoon finely chopped dill, plus extra to serve
1 tablespoon balsamic vinegar
3 spring onions, sliced
salt and pepper

1. Preheat the oven to 200°C/180°C fan (400°F), Gas Mark 6.
2. Put the potatoes in a medium-sized roasting tray (mine measured 34 × 24cm/13½ × 9½ inches), spray with spray oil and season with salt and pepper. Place on the middle shelf of the oven for 20 minutes.
3. Make up the coating for the pork by mixing the lemon zest, yogurt, garlic and some salt and pepper in a bowl.
4. Remove the tray of potatoes from the oven, place the pork tenderloin into the middle of the tray (shuffling the potatoes to the sides), and spread the yogurt mixture over the meat. Sprinkle a little bit of paprika over the top of this and return to the oven for 10 minutes.
5. Remove the tray from the oven, scatter the beetroot among the potatoes, spray with a little more oil, increase the oven temperature to 220°C/200°C fan (425°F), Gas Mark 7 and roast for a final 10 minutes.
6. Check the pork is cooked. Pork tenderloins can vary in thickness, so you will need to check that it is cooked through at its thickest part before serving. If you have a meat thermometer, it should read at least 75°C (167°F). Lift it on to a chopping board to rest for 5 minutes. Meanwhile, add the dill, balsamic vinegar and spring onions to the potatoes and beetroot and stir them in.
7. Slice the pork thinly, then serve the potato and beetroot and top with the pork. Sprinkle with extra dill to serve.

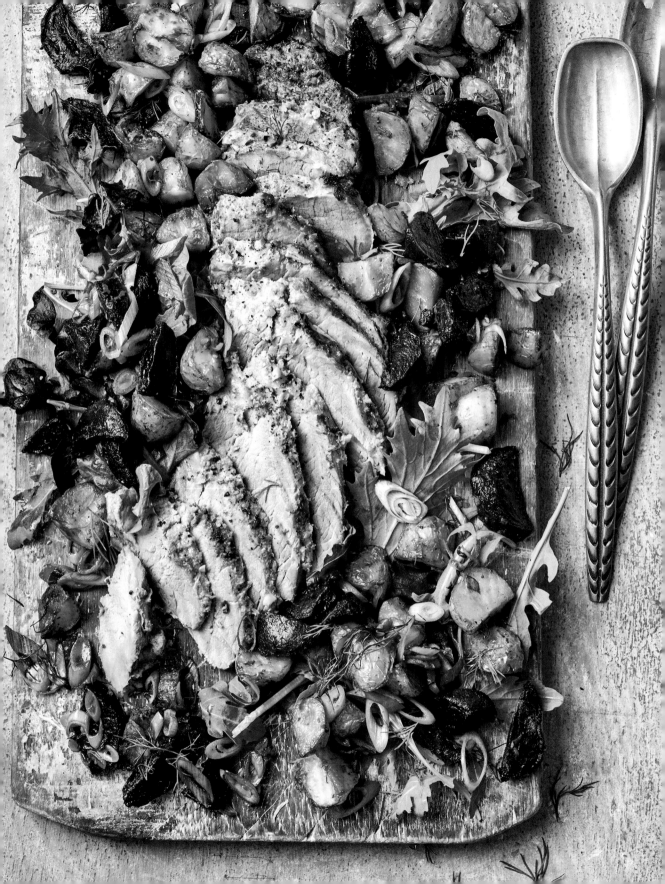

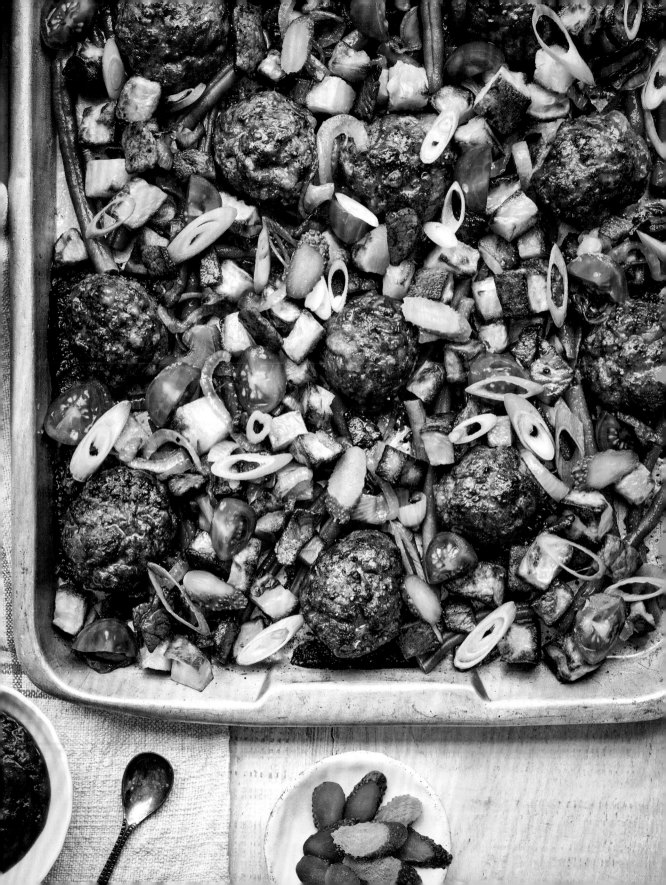

SERVES 4

CHEESEBURGER BALLS
WITH LOADED CHIPPIES

Classic cheeseburger flavours all wrapped up in meatballs, with little
roasted potato cubes (we call them chippies in our house!) loaded up
with onions, bacon and roasted green beans. A healthier alternative to
a cheeseburger, and just as satisfying.

CALORIES PER SERVING: 502
PREP TIME: 20 MINUTES
COOK TIME: 40 MINUTES

800g (1lb 12oz) potatoes, peeled
   and cut into 1cm (½ inch) cubes
1 teaspoon olive oil
500g (1lb 2oz) minced beef (less
   than 5 per cent fat)
1 tablespoon American mustard
1 tablespoon oyster sauce
1 tablespoon tomato ketchup
1 tablespoon mixed herbs
1 teaspoon onion granules
1 teaspoon garlic granules
½ teaspoon salt
¼ teaspoon pepper
60g (2¼oz) red Leicester cheese,
   grated
2 onions, sliced
200g (7oz) green beans, trimmed
2 smoked bacon medallions,
   finely chopped
low-calorie cooking spray
3 spring onions, sliced
100g (3½oz) cherry tomatoes,
   quartered
gherkins, sliced, to serve
   (optional)
coarse sea salt and pepper

1. Preheat the oven to 220°C/200°C fan (425°F), Gas Mark 7.
2. In an extra-large baking tray (mine measured 38 × 30cm/15 × 12 inches), coat the potato cubes in the oil and season them with a few grinds of coarse sea salt, then pop them into the oven for 20 minutes.
3. In a large bowl, mix together the beef, mustard, oyster sauce, tomato ketchup, mixed herbs, onion granules, garlic granules, measured salt and pepper and red Leicester. Form this mix into 12 large meatballs.
4. Remove the potatoes from the oven and stir in the onions, green beans and bacon. Place the meatballs amongst the vegetables, season and then give everything a spray with low-calorie cooking spray. Roast for 20 minutes.
5. Scatter with spring onions, cherry tomatoes and gherkins (if using) and serve.

NOTE Load these up with your favourite toppings, you could add mushrooms, peppers, asparagus or pepperoni in step 4, or load on toppings when serving, such as roasted red peppers, jalapeños, crisp shredded lettuce, extra cheese or spring onions.

BAKED MAPLE ALMOND RICE PUDDING

My childhood rice puddings were always baked in the oven and had a crust on top. This is a light version of a baked rice pudding, using almond milk and complemented with sweet maple syrup, slivers of caramelized orange zest and crunchy flaked almonds, which makes a great 'Sunday dinner' pudding. It is delicious on its own, or served with a dollop of jam. Pudding rice is fairly widely available in supermarkets, usually in the same aisle as canned rice pudding.

CALORIES PER SERVING: 170
PREP TIME: 5 MINUTES
COOK TIME: 1 HOUR 25 MINUTES

150g (5½oz) pudding rice
1 litre (1¾ pints) unsweetened almond milk
3 tablespoons pure maple syrup
1 teaspoon vanilla extract
1 unwaxed orange
1 tablespoon dark brown muscovado sugar, plus extra to serve (optional)
2 tablespoons flaked almonds
salt

1. Preheat the oven to 150°C/130°C fan (300°F), Gas Mark 2.
2. In a baking dish (mine was 24 × 19cm/9½ × 7½ inches), mix together the rice, almond milk, maple syrup, vanilla and a pinch of salt. Try to make sure that the rice is evenly spread out.
3. To zest the orange, use a sharp potato peeler to peel off 1–2cm (½–¾ inch) slivers of the top layer of zest. Try to avoid taking off the white pith underneath. Zest half the orange, then place the slivers evenly around the top of the rice.
4. Place on to the middle shelf of the oven and bake for 1 hour.
5. After an hour, increase the oven temperature to 200°C/180°C fan (400°F), Gas Mark 6. Sprinkle the sugar and then the flaked almonds over the top (a skin will have started to form), then return the dish to the oven for another 25 minutes. By this time the rice should be cooked through, will have absorbed the milk and formed a light golden crust over the top.
6. If liked, sprinkle over a little bit of dark brown sugar and finely grated orange zest.

NOTE For a slightly more indulgent (and delicious) version, add a few blobs of almond butter on the top of the rice in step 3 and swirl them through before adding the orange zest.

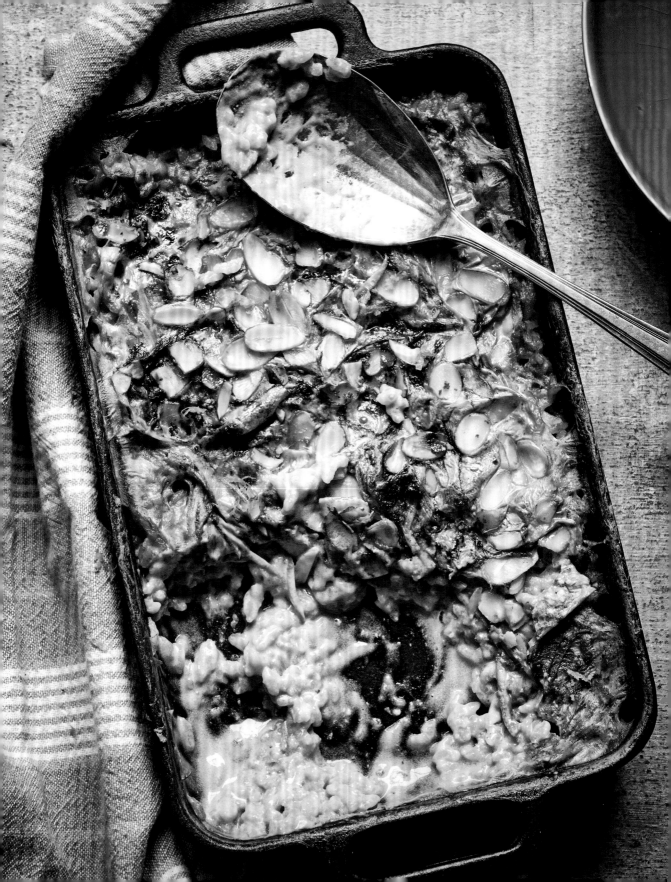

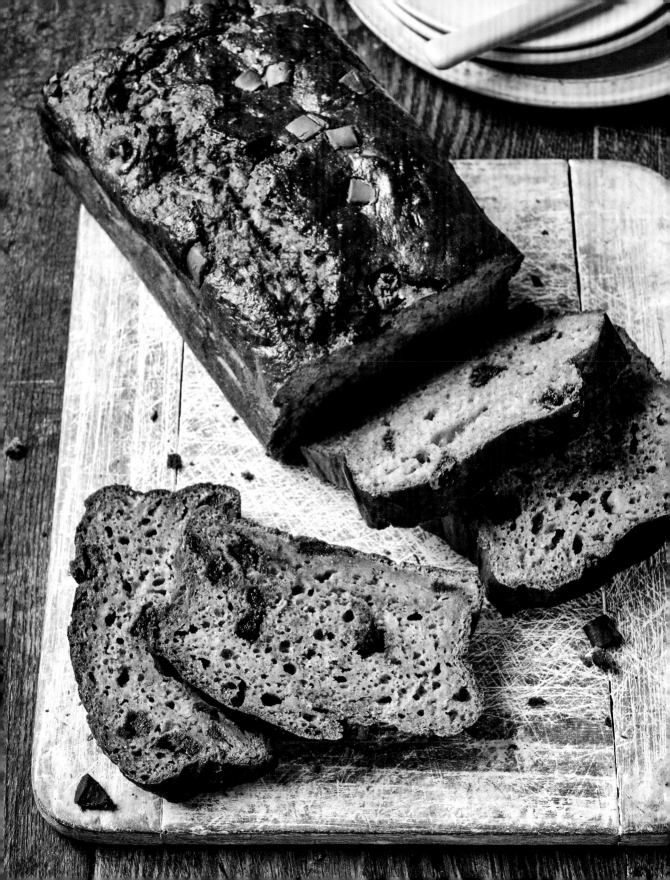

NEVER BORING BANANA BREAD

I always find it a tricky balance to produce a 'healthy' cake; generally, it's hard to make it taste great without using the more indulgent ingredients. My approach is to try to make bakes as healthy as possible, but enough of a treat that everyone still wants to eat them. So I have made this largely with wholemeal flour, to increase the fibre content, cut down on the sugar and used yogurt instead of butter, margarine or oil. It received my 11-year-old's seal of approval and I gave in to her insistence that banana bread should always include chocolate chips!

CALORIES PER SERVING: 166
PREP TIME: 10 MINUTES,
PLUS COOLING TIME
COOK TIME: 50 MINUTES

3 small ripe bananas (approx. 225g/8oz peeled weight)

2 large eggs, lightly beaten

4 tablespoons pure maple syrup

2 tablespoons light soft brown sugar

150g (5½oz) fat-free Greek yogurt

1 teaspoon vanilla extract

1 teaspoon ground cinnamon

¼ teaspoon salt

2 teaspoons baking powder

150g (5½oz) plain wholemeal flour (not wholemeal bread flour)

90g (3¼oz) white self-raising flour

50g (1¾oz) milk or dark chocolate chips

low-calorie cooking spray

1. Preheat the oven to 180°C/160°C fan (350°F), Gas Mark 4.
2. In a large mixing bowl, mash the bananas with a fork, then mix in the eggs, maple syrup and sugar. Stir in the yogurt, vanilla, cinnamon, salt and baking powder.
3. Stir in the flours with a wooden spoon to form a batter, then stir in the chocolate chips.
4. Line a 900g (2lb) loaf tin with baking paper or a loaf tin liner and spray with low-calorie cooking spray. Spoon the batter into the tin and spread out evenly.
5. Bake on the bottom shelf of the oven for 50 minutes. The loaf will rise (and the top may crack) and will be well browned on top. Insert a knife to make sure that it is cooked through: if the knife comes out clean, it is done; if it comes out covered in batter, you will need to bake it for longer.
6. Allow to cool slightly and serve warm.

NOTE This cake is at its best warm but keeps well in an airtight container in a cool place for about 4 days (allow it to fully cool before transferring into a sealed container). One of our favourite ways to eat it in the days after baking is toasted and spread with peanut butter, almond butter or chocolate spread. The banana bread is also delicious with walnuts or pecans added.

RASPBERRY & PISTACHIO TRAYCAKE

This is effectively one big old pancake, cooked in the oven. I have been making oat-based pancakes for years, and they are a great way to have a healthier version of a traditional pancake. It is a quick, easy, hands-off recipe, as there is no standing over a pan. Pistachios add delicious flavour as well as lovely little specks of green which look so appealing. I have said this serves 4, as I find it is filling enough for breakfast with berries and yogurt. I like a drizzle of maple syrup over the top as well to add sweetness (as there is nothing sweet other than raspberries in the batter).

CALORIES PER SERVING: 178
PREP TIME: 5 MINUTES
COOK TIME: 15 MINUTES

80g (2¾oz) porridge oats
20 shelled and unsalted
    pistachios
1 teaspoon baking powder
¼ teaspoon ground cinnamon
2 large eggs
150g (5½oz) fat-free Greek
    yogurt, plus extra to serve
1 teaspoon vanilla extract
low-calorie cooking spray
100g (3½oz) frozen raspberries,
    crushed into small bits
salt

TO SERVE
pure maple syrup
fresh berries
yogurt

1. Preheat the oven to 200°C/180°C fan (400°F), Gas Mark 6.
2. In a food processor, blend together the oats, pistachios, baking powder and cinnamon until the oats are almost a flour and the pistachios are finely chopped. Add the eggs, yogurt, vanilla and a pinch of salt to the food processor bowl and whizz to form a batter.
3. Line a small baking tray (about 26 × 20cm/10½ × 8 inches) with baking parchment and spray with low-calorie cooking spray. Pour the batter into the lined tray and spread it out evenly with a spatula.
4. Scatter the berry pieces evenly over the top and spray with low-calorie cooking spray.
5. Bake for 15 minutes. After this time the traycake should be cooked through and golden brown on top.
6. Serve with a drizzle of maple syrup, fresh berries and a dollop of yogurt.

NOTE You can mix up the flavour combinations here – try different nuts such as hazelnuts, cashews, peanuts and almonds, and different fruit such as blueberries, blackberries or banana. If you fancy a little bit of extra indulgence, throw a small handful of white chocolate chips into the mix.

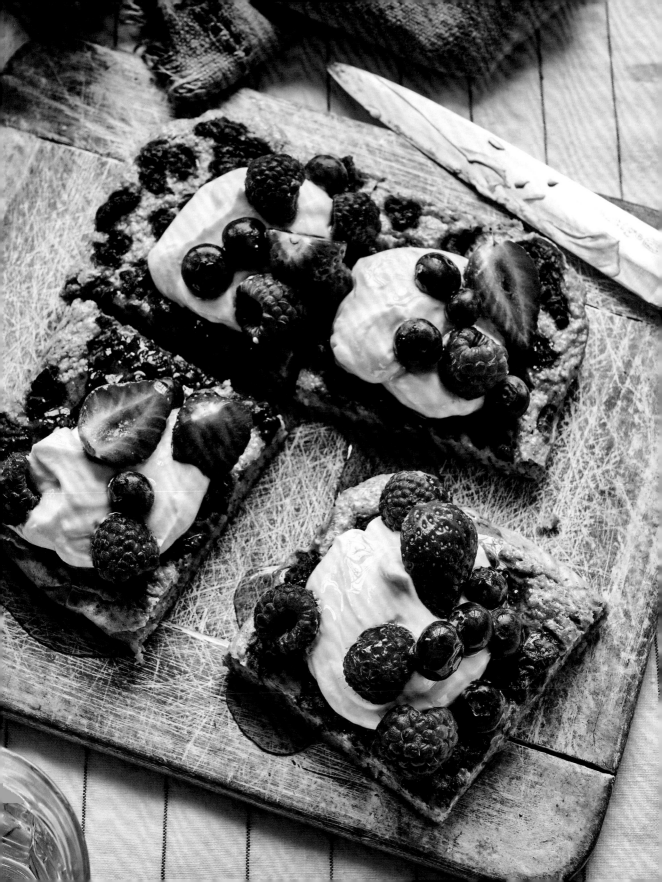

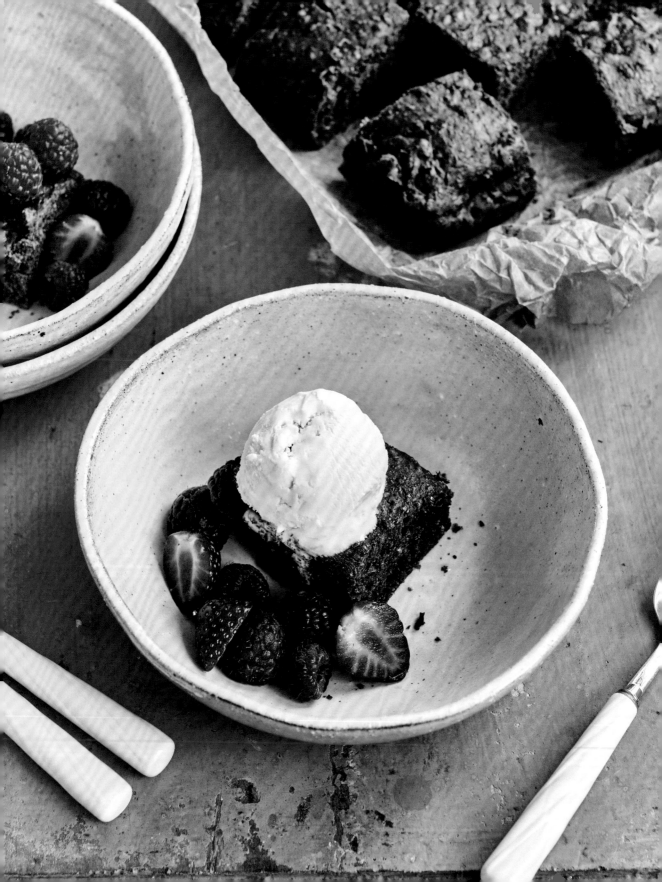

SERVES 16

HEALTHIER CHOCOLATE CAKE

**Who doesn't love a warm piece of freshly baked chocolate cake?
It is the bake most requested by my children and over the years I have
gradually tweaked a classic recipe to make it just a little more healthy.
This recipe mixes wholemeal and white flour to get a bit of fibre in,
combines butter with fat-free yogurt to reduce the fat content and
uses a reduced amount of sugar, but enough that it still tastes good.
It all gets wolfed down!**

CALORIES PER SERVING: 107
PREP TIME: 10 MINUTES
COOK TIME: 20 MINUTES

100g (3½oz) fat-free Greek
    yogurt
50g (1¾oz) salted butter,
    softened
3 large eggs
100g (3½oz) light soft brown
    sugar
3 teaspoons vanilla extract
1 teaspoon baking powder
30g (1oz) cocoa powder
100g (3½oz) plain wholemeal
    flour
50g (1¾oz) white self-raising
    flour

1. Preheat the oven to 200°C/180°C fan (400°F), Gas Mark 6.
2. In a large bowl, mix together the yogurt, butter, eggs, sugar and vanilla. Add the baking powder, cocoa powder and both flours and use a wooden spoon to mix it into a smooth batter.
3. Line a square (23cm/9 inch) cake tin with baking paper and pour in all the batter, then smooth over the top.
4. Bake on the middle shelf of the oven for 20 minutes.
5. Allow to cool in the tin for 5-10 minutes, before removing from the tin and cutting into portions. Store in an airtight container for 3-4 days at room temperature, or up to 5 days in the refrigerator.

NOTE Because of the wholemeal flour, once this cake cools, it has a slightly harder consistency than regular chocolate cake. My family are perfectly happy with this, but you can always warm it up in a microwave to bring it back to the full, freshly baked experience! For a dessert, serve this warm with fresh raspberries and strawberries and vanilla ice cream, if you like.

CHAPTER 4

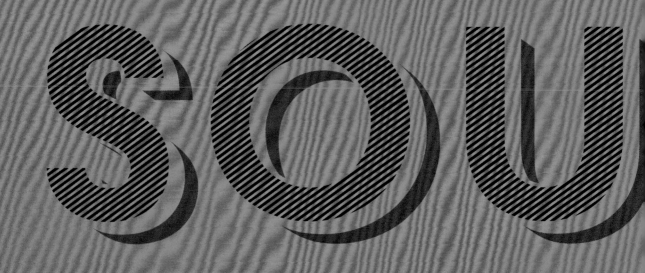

P-ER

SPICED TOMATO, LENTIL & CHICKPEA SOUP

A soup so thick and hearty that it is almost a stew. Packed with nutritious ingredients, it's ideal for a filling lunch with friends. I serve it with warm pitta bread (see my Wholemeal Pitta Bread on page 202).

CALORIES PER SERVING: 246
PREP TIME: 15 MINUTES
COOK TIME: 1 HOUR

2 onions, quartered
2 celery sticks, roughly chopped
1 teaspoon olive oil
400g (14oz) can of plum tomatoes
2 carrots, peeled and roughly chopped
4 garlic cloves
large handful of parsley leaves, plus extra, chopped, to serve
1 red chilli, deseeded and finely chopped
1 litre (1¾ pints) hot vegetable stock
150g (5½oz) dried red lentils
400g (14oz) can of chickpeas, drained and rinsed
1 sweet potato, peeled and chopped
3 tablespoons tomato purée
2 lemons, cut into wedges, to serve

FOR THE SPICE MIX
1 teaspoon ground cumin
1 teaspoon ground turmeric
1 teaspoon ground ginger
½ teaspoon ground cinnamon
½ teaspoon salt
½ teaspoon pepper

1. Make up the spice mix in a small bowl by stirring together all the ingredients.
2. In a food processor, blend the onions and celery until very finely chopped.
3. In a large saucepan, heat the oil and scrape in the onion and celery. Fry gently for 10 minutes, stirring every now and again to prevent sticking. Meanwhile, put the tomatoes, carrots, garlic, parsley and chilli in the food processor and blend until smooth.
4. After 10 minutes, increase the heat, add the spice blend to the onions and celery and stir through for 30 seconds. Reduce the heat to low and pour in the tomato mixture. Stir through, then add the hot stock, red lentils, chickpeas, sweet potato and tomato purée.
5. Bring to the boil, then reduce the heat and gently simmer for 45 minutes, stirring occasionally. Serve with lemon wedges and parsley.

NOTE If I have leftovers of my slow-cooker Fakeaway Doner Kebab (see page 169), I chop them up and throw them into this soup for a delicious meaty option. If you have coriander or mint leaves to use up, they are also a great addition to this meal.

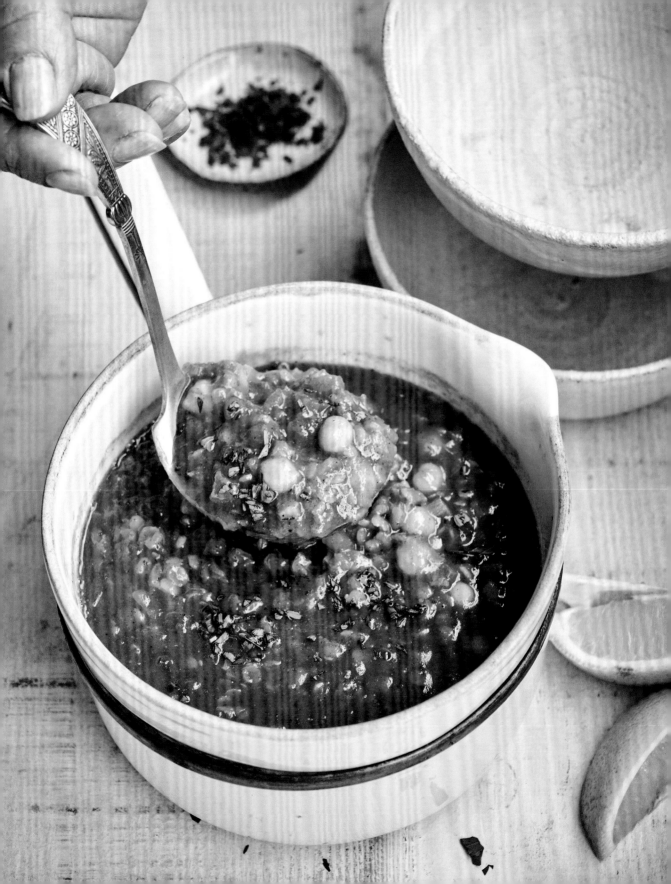

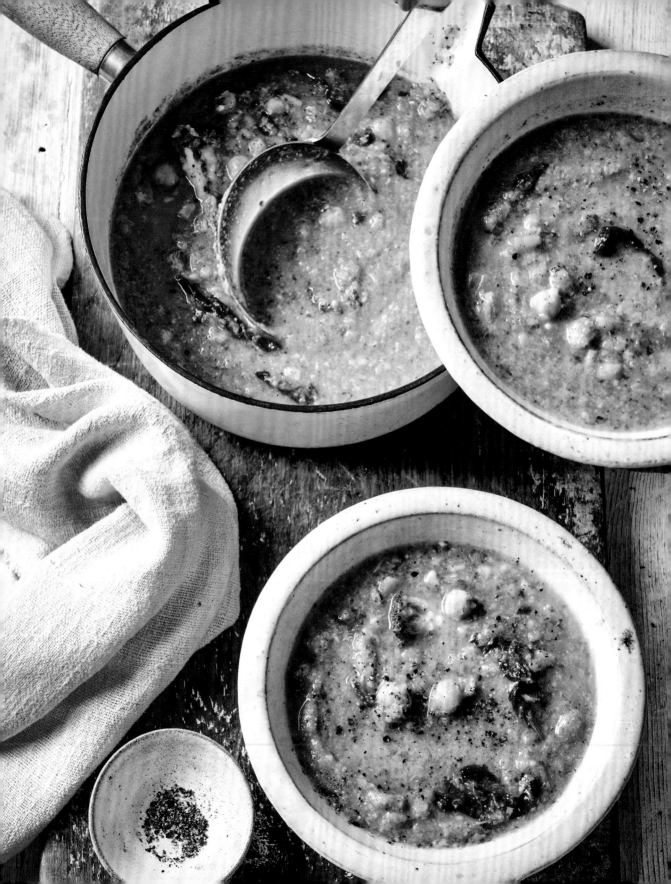

SUPER-GREEN SOUP

**This is the soup for a real vitamin boost! The chickpeas give
it extra filling power and fibre to help keep you fuller for longer,
while the addition of fennel adds a subtle flavour which makes
it both delicious and healthy.**

CALORIES PER SERVING: 142
PREP TIME: 20 MINUTES
COOK TIME: 30 MINUTES

spray oil
2 onions, finely chopped
2 celery sticks, finely chopped
1 fennel bulb, trimmed and
    sliced (see box below)
2 garlic cloves, finely chopped
2 courgettes, roughly chopped
1 head of broccoli, florets cut
    away, stalk trimmed and
    chopped (see box below)
1 litre (1¾ pints) hot vegetable
    stock
400g (14oz) can of chickpeas,
    drained and rinsed
small handful of parsley leaves
2 large handfuls of baby spinach
juice of 1 lemon
salt and pepper

1. Spray some oil into a large, deep casserole dish (with a lid) and fry the onions and celery over a medium heat for 5 minutes, stirring occasionally. Add the fennel, garlic, courgettes and broccoli stalks and fry gently for 10 minutes, stirring every now and again so nothing gets stuck to the bottom of the pan.
2. Pour in the hot stock and add the chickpeas, bring to the boil and cook at a fast simmer for 5 minutes.
3. Add the broccoli florets, parsley and spinach, pop a lid on the pan and allow to simmer for 7–8 minutes, until the broccoli is tender.
4. Season with salt and pepper, squeeze in the lemon juice and use a hand blender to blend it into a smooth soup, or leave it chunkier if you prefer.

HOW TO PREPARE FENNEL
Cut away the shoots from the top of the fennel, cut off the root, then remove and discard the tough outer leaves. Cut the fennel lengthways down the centre, then slice finely across the bulb as you would with an onion.

HOW TO PREPARE BROCCOLI STALKS
Don't throw away your broccoli stalks! Simply use a sharp knife to trim away the very tough outer bits and the base of the stalk, then slice into coins or matchsticks to add to the soup.

SERVES 2

HOT & SOUR MUSHROOM NOODLE SOUP

This is a quick and flavour-packed soup which is satisfyingly sweet and sour and full of comforting chilli warmth. Tamarind paste is a really useful ingredient to keep on hand at home for adding rich flavour to a variety of dishes. You can use fine or medium egg noodles instead of the instant packet ramen noodles.

CALORIES PER SERVING: 264
PREP TIME: 5 MINUTES
COOK TIME: 12 MINUTES

spray oil
1 onion, finely chopped
2 garlic cloves, crushed
1 red chilli, deseeded and finely
    chopped
250g (9oz) chestnut
    mushrooms, sliced
750ml (1 pint 7fl oz) hot
    vegetable stock
1 tablespoon tamarind paste
1 tablespoon dark soy sauce
1 teaspoon honey
1 packet instant ramen noodles
    (flavour sachet not used)
coriander leaves, to serve

1. In a deep saucepan, fry the onion gently in spray oil for 5 minutes.
2. Add the garlic, chilli and mushrooms and fry gently for another 5 minutes.
3. Pour in the hot stock, add the tamarind paste, soy sauce and honey and stir well.
4. Add the instant noodles to the pot and simmer for 2 minutes until the noodles are cooked. Serve immediately, scattered with fresh coriander.

MAGIC RAMEN
Instant ramen noodles are a great ingredient to have on hand for quick noodle soups, as they only take 2 minutes to rehydrate. I usually don't use the flavour sachets that come with them. You can also crush the noodles up and use them as a crunchy textured topping for salads, or even as a breadcrumb replacement to make a crispy coating for baked chicken or fish.

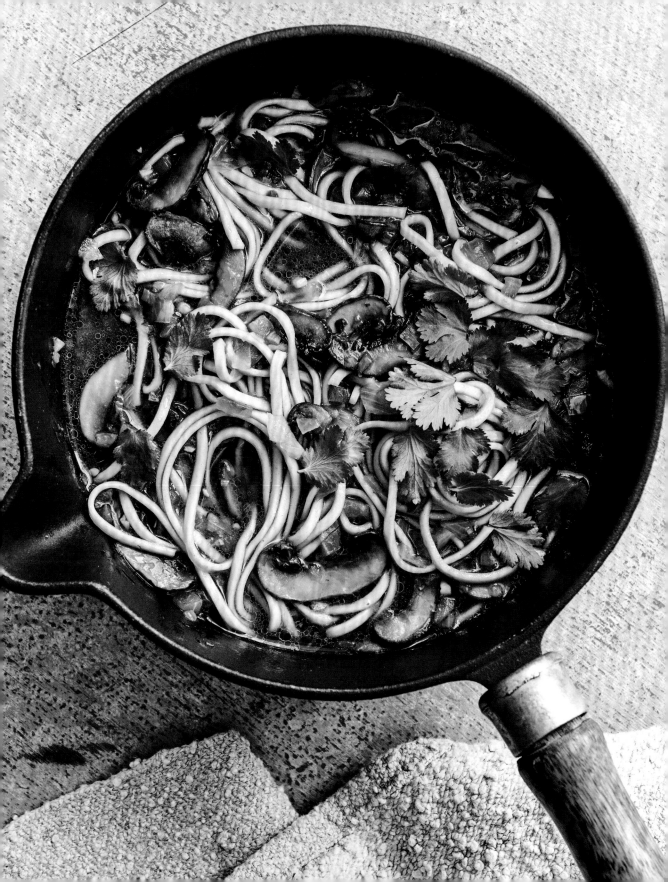

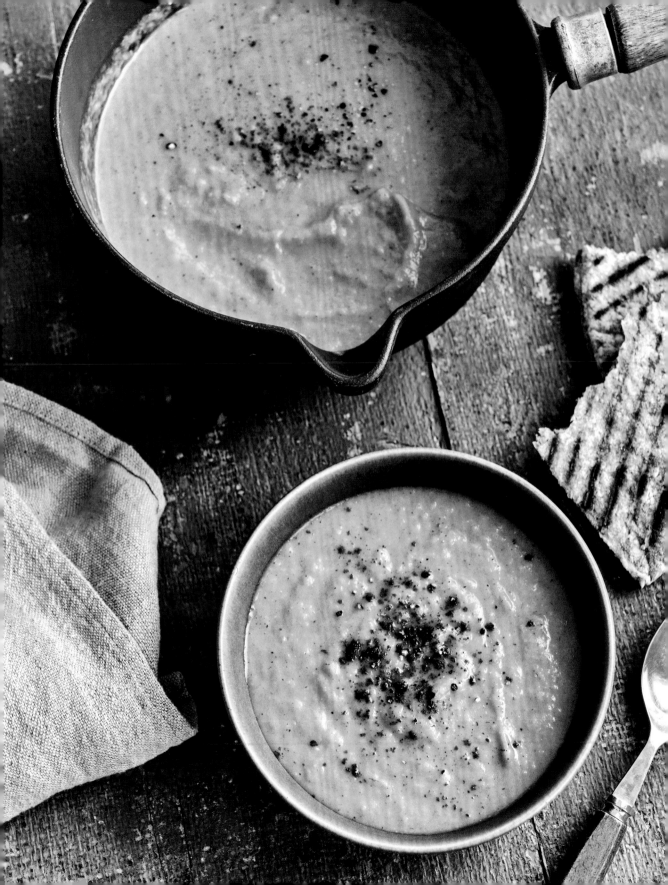

SERVES 4

SPICED LEEK & POTATO SOUP

Take a simple leek and potato soup to a new level with some warming spices: lovely, nutritious comfort food. I like to eat this with warm pitta bread (for my Wholemeal Pitta Bread recipe, see page 202).

CALORIES PER SERVING: 129
PREP TIME: 10 MINUTES
COOK TIME: 35 MINUTES

spray oil
1 large onion, finely chopped
4 medium leeks, trimmed and
    sliced
2 medium potatoes, peeled and
    finely chopped
1 garlic clove, crushed
½ teaspoon ground cumin
½ teaspoon ground ginger
½ teaspoon ground turmeric
1 teaspoon salt
750ml (1 pint 7fl oz) hot
    vegetable stock

TO SERVE
sprinkling of smoked paprika
pepper

1. Spray a large saucepan with oil and fry the onion, leeks and potatoes over a high heat for 2 minutes.
2. Stir in the garlic, reduce the heat to low, pop the lid on the pan and leave it gently sizzling and sweating for 15 minutes, stirring it halfway through to prevent any sticking.
3. Remove the lid, increase the heat, add the spices and salt and stir through for about 30 seconds until you can smell the spices. Pour in the hot stock and allow to simmer for 15 minutes.
4. Use a hand blender to blend the soup to a smooth consistency.
5. Serve sprinkled with a little smoked paprika, just for a pop of colour, and pepper.

ARRABBIATA ORZO SOUP

A very simple, quick-to-make tomato soup based on a traditional Italian arrabbiatta sauce (tomato, chilli and garlic). I like to make this when I have very little time for prepping, but want something filling and warming for lunch. I love orzo in soup because, as well as thickening it up, it adds great texture and filling power.

CALORIES PER SERVING: 243
PREP TIME: 5 MINUTES
COOK TIME: 20 MINUTES

5 garlic cloves
1 teaspoon chilli flakes
2 × 400g (14oz) cans of chopped
   tomatoes
500ml (18fl oz) hot vegetable
   stock
1 teaspoon salt
½ teaspoon pepper, plus extra
   to serve
200g (7oz) orzo

TO SERVE
basil leaves
Parmesan-style vegetarian
   cheese, grated

1. Put the garlic, chilli and tomatoes in a food processor and whizz until completely smooth.
2. Pour the tomato mixture into a large saucepan, add the vegetable stock, salt and pepper and bring up to a fast simmer.
3. Add the orzo and simmer for 15–20 minutes until the orzo is cooked through, stirring regularly to ensure that it doesn't stick to the bottom of the pan.
4. Serve with basil leaves, a scattering of grated cheese and a few grinds of black pepper.

NOTE The starch in the pasta can make this quite thick. If you prefer a more pourable consistency, add extra vegetable stock (just check that the seasoning levels are still right), or cook the orzo separately and add it at the end. I also sometimes like to blend fresh herbs (basil, oregano or parsley) into the tomato sauce in step 1 for extra herby flavour.

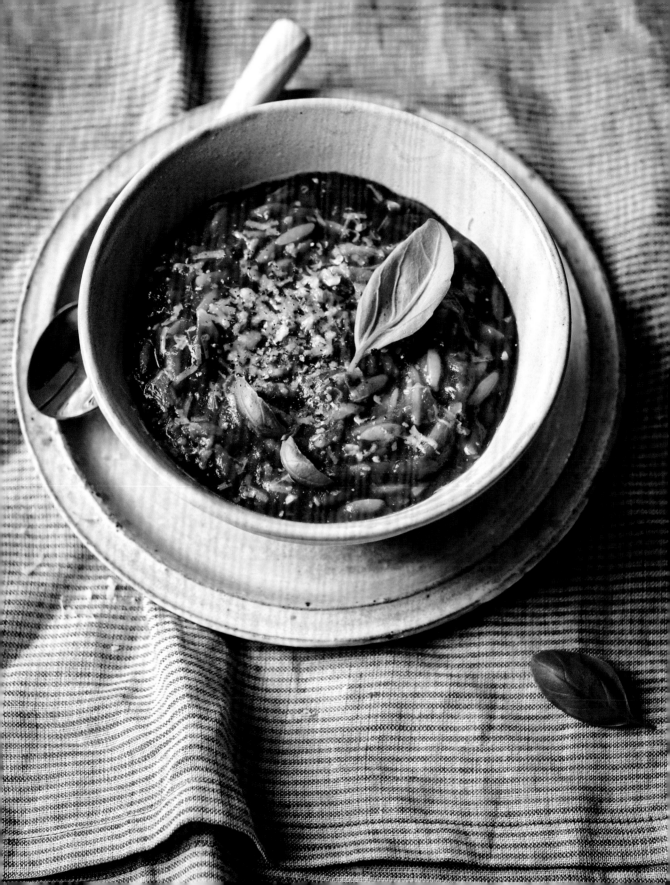

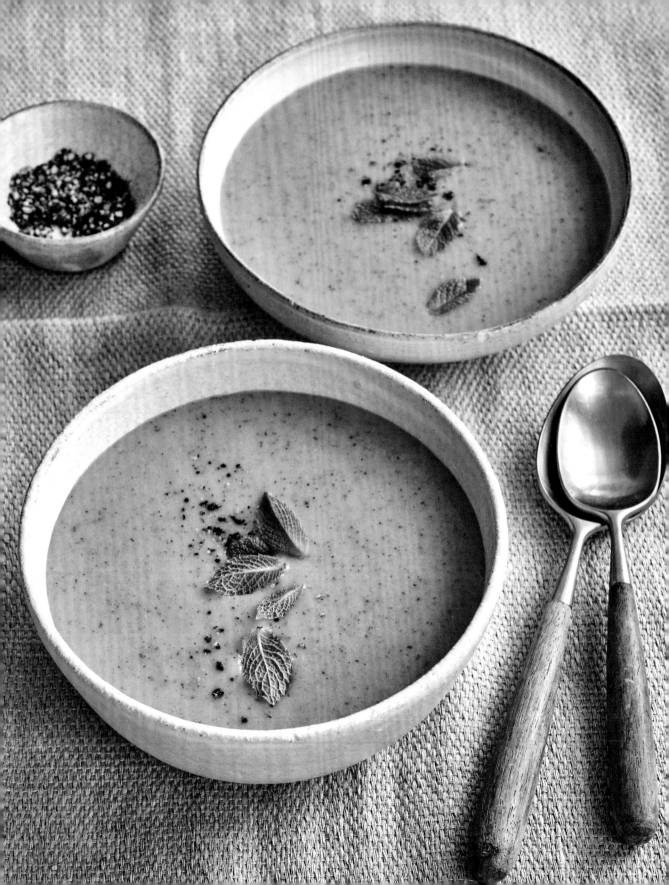

COURGETTE, CANNELLINI, PEA & MINT SOUP

A summery, refreshing soup with flavours of pea and mint, but with the filling power of cannellini beans, blended in for a thick consistency.

CALORIES PER SERVING: 94
PREP TIME: 10 MINUTES
COOK TIME: 25 MINUTES

spray oil
1 onion, finely chopped
2 courgettes, roughly chopped
2 garlic cloves, crushed
750ml (1 pint 7fl oz) hot
    vegetable stock
400g (14oz) can of cannellini
    beans, drained and rinsed
200g (7oz) frozen peas,
    defrosted
large handful of mint leaves,
    plus extra to serve
salt and pepper

1. Spray a large saucepan with oil and fry the onion, courgettes and garlic for 10 minutes over a gentle heat.
2. Pour in the hot stock, add the cannellini beans and peas and simmer for 15 minutes.
3. Remove from the heat, add the mint leaves, season with salt and pepper and use a hand blender to blend the soup to a smooth consistency.
4. Serve with extra mint leaves and grind over some pepper.

GROW YOUR OWN

I use a lot of mint in my cooking, partly because I always have it readily available. Mint is one of those herbs that is so easy to grow that you don't need to do any work to keep an impressive crop. I'm not a gardener by any stretch, but I love that I can always pop out for mint (and I kept it on the windowsill before I had a garden). Mint is best grown in a large pot, as it can take over flower beds very quickly. Use a multi-purpose compost and, if you are using a plant from the supermarket or garden centre to start with, tip it gently out of the pot it came in and carefully split it apart at the roots into 2–3 parts which you can plant spaced out in its destination pot. As you pick it, new leaves will quickly grow, or you can keep 2 pots and alternate which plant you pick from to keep a constant supply.

LEEK, LENTIL & ORZO POTAGE

Potage is a thick soup and this version is packed full of tasty vegetables and thickened with lentils and orzo for a thoroughly filling and nutritious bowl of goodness. Taking a little time chopping all the vegetables pays off, as this tastes great reheated and makes an ideal lunch on-the-go in a soup flask.

CALORIES PER SERVING: 208
PREP TIME: 20 MINUTES
COOK TIME: 30 MINUTES

spray oil
150g (5½oz) cherry tomatoes, halved
3 shallots, finely chopped
2 garlic cloves, crushed
1 celery stick, finely chopped
1 fennel bulb, trimmed and finely chopped (see page 137)
1 leek, trimmed and finely chopped
800ml (1 pint 8fl oz) hot vegetable stock
100g (3½oz) orzo
400g (14oz) can of green lentils, drained and rinsed
1 courgette, finely chopped
small handful of basil leaves, finely chopped, plus extra to serve
salt and pepper

1. Spray a casserole dish or deep saucepan with oil and stir-fry the tomatoes over a high heat for 2 minutes.
2. Add the shallots and garlic to the pan and fry for a further 3 minutes.
3. Add the celery, fennel and leek to the pan, stir everything through and fry for another 5 minutes over a medium heat, stirring occasionally to prevent anything from sticking to the bottom of the pan.
4. Pour in the hot stock, add the orzo, lentils and courgette and allow to simmer gently for 15–20 minutes until the orzo is cooked through.
5. Season to taste with salt and pepper, stir through most of the chopped basil and serve with a little more basil scattered over the top.

NOTE If you would like to keep this pasta-free, just omit the orzo. You can add additional flavour if you fancy by stirring through 1 teaspoon of pesto or harissa paste. If you have leftover fennel, try the Super-Green Soup (see page 137).

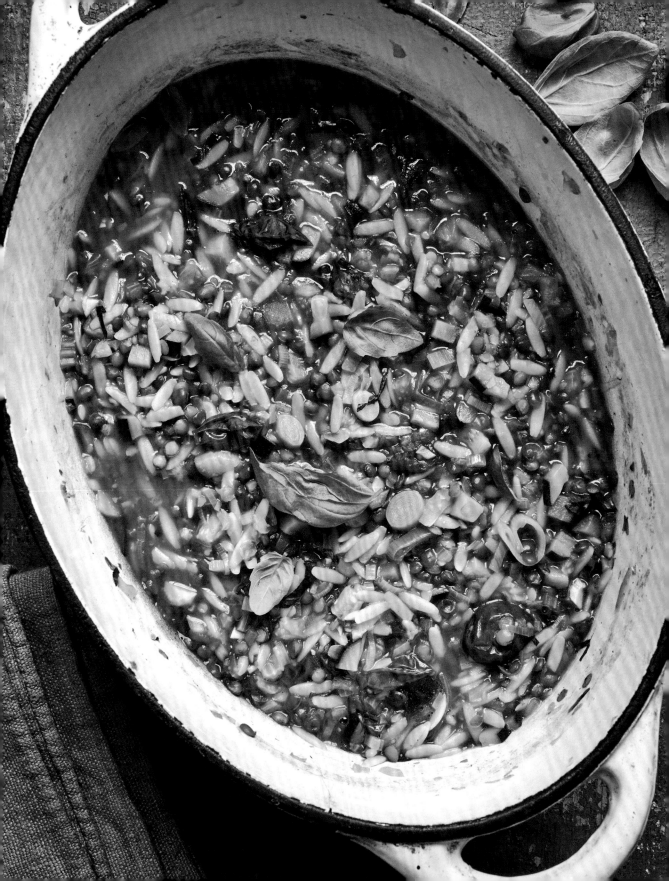

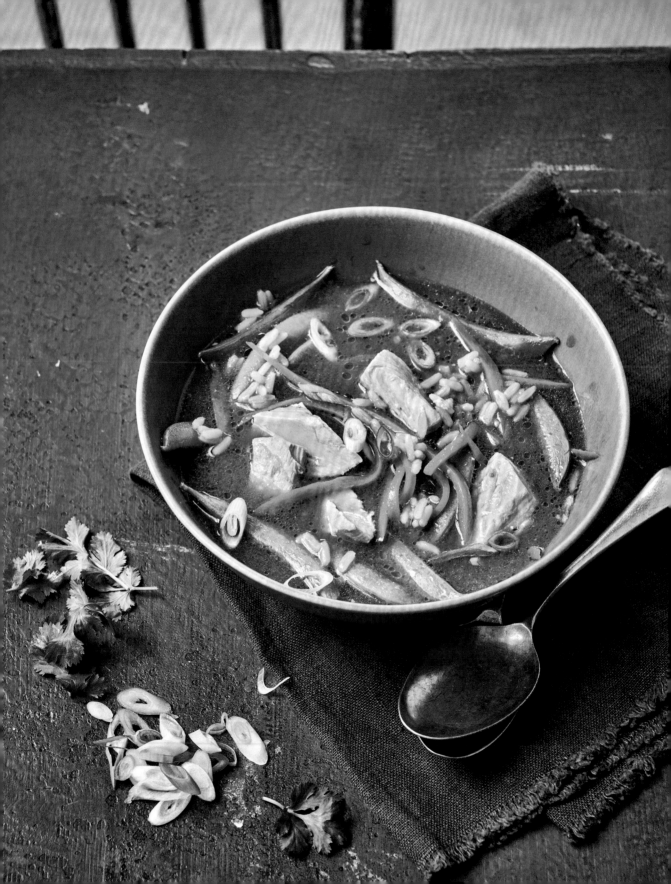

SERVES 2

SALMON & MISO BROTH

For a quick lunch or a light supper, this Japanese-inspired soup ticks all the boxes. It only takes 5 minutes to prepare and 12 minutes to cook. The miso paste and mirin are a magical combination that give both savoury and sweet flavours, marrying so perfectly with delicately poached chunks of salmon and crunchy sugarsnap peas. Most big supermarkets will sell both miso paste and mirin near the soy sauce and noodles and they are both really useful ingredients to have in stock.

CALORIES PER SERVING: 519
PREP TIME: 5 MINUTES
COOK TIME: 12 MINUTES

500ml (18fl oz) chicken stock
50g (1¾oz) long grain rice
1 tablespoon miso paste
1 tablespoon mirin
1 tablespoon light soy sauce
2 carrots, peeled and cut into
    fine matchsticks
2 salmon fillets, skin removed,
    cut into bite-sized chunks
75g (2¾oz) sugarsnap peas

TO SERVE (OPTIONAL)
chopped spring onions
coriander leaves

1. In a medium-sized saucepan, bring the stock to the boil, add the rice and simmer for 7 minutes.
2. Add the miso paste to the pan and stir to dissolve, then add the mirin, soy sauce, carrots and salmon.
3. Simmer for 3 minutes, add the sugarsnap peas, then simmer for another 2 minutes.
4. Serve just as it is, or with some spring onions and coriander scattered over.

WHAT IS MISO?
Miso is a fermented soy bean paste and a common Japanese ingredient. It has a distinctive salty, umami (which roughly translates to 'deliciousness' in Japanese) flavour.

WHAT IS MIRIN?
Mirin is a Japanese sweet rice cooking wine. Offering both sweet and umami tastes, it can add amazing flavour to marinades, sauces, soups, stir-fries and salad dressings.

CHICKEN & PRAWN LAKSA

My version of laksa is pretty simplified, but still packs a real flavour punch without being too complicated to put together.

CALORIES PER SERVING: 526
PREP TIME: 15 MINUTES
COOK TIME: 30 MINUTES

spray oil
800ml (1 pint 8fl oz) hot chicken
   stock
400ml (14fl oz) can of light coconut
   milk
2 tablespoons sweet chilli sauce
finely grated zest and juice of
   1 unwaxed lime
½ teaspoon ground turmeric
2–3 chicken breasts (total weight
   about 400g/14oz), chopped small
200g (7oz) cooked peeled cold-
   water prawns
200g (7oz) medium egg noodles
200g (7oz) beansprouts
salt

FOR THE LAKSA PASTE
1 red chilli, deseeded
1 lemon grass stalk, trimmed and
   roughly chopped (see box below)
2 garlic cloves
2.5cm (1 inch) piece of fresh root
   ginger, peeled
1 tablespoon fish sauce
40g (1½oz) flaked almonds
2 spring onions, roughly chopped
2 tablespoons water

TO SERVE
coriander leaves
lime wedges

1. Put all the paste ingredients into a mini chopper and blend until smooth.
2. I use a large, nonstick casserole dish to make this. Use spray oil to fry the paste gently for 2 minutes, then add the hot stock, coconut milk, sweet chilli sauce, lime zest and juice and turmeric.
3. Bring to the boil, add the chicken, then reduce to a simmer and cook for 20 minutes.
4. Add the prawns and noodles (make sure the noodles are submerged) and simmer for a further 5 minutes, or until the noodles are cooked through.
5. Stir in the beansprouts, season to taste with salt, and serve scattered with coriander leaves and with a lime wedge on the side.

NOTE You can use your noodles of choice in this: thicker noodles work well, or rice noodles. If I'm making it for my children, I omit the chilli from the paste and add some chilli sauce to mine when I serve it up. I also usually add a few baby sweetcorns for them, in step 4 with the noodles and prawns.

> ### HOW TO PREPARE LEMON GRASS
> Start by using a sharp knife to slice away the base and tip, then remove the really tough, woody outer leaves by hand, leaving the softer yellow fleshy part. Thinly slice to about two-thirds of the way up the stalk. You can save the tough top part for flavouring curries or soups - just give it a bit of a bash to help release the oils and throw into the pot. Remember to fish it out before serving!

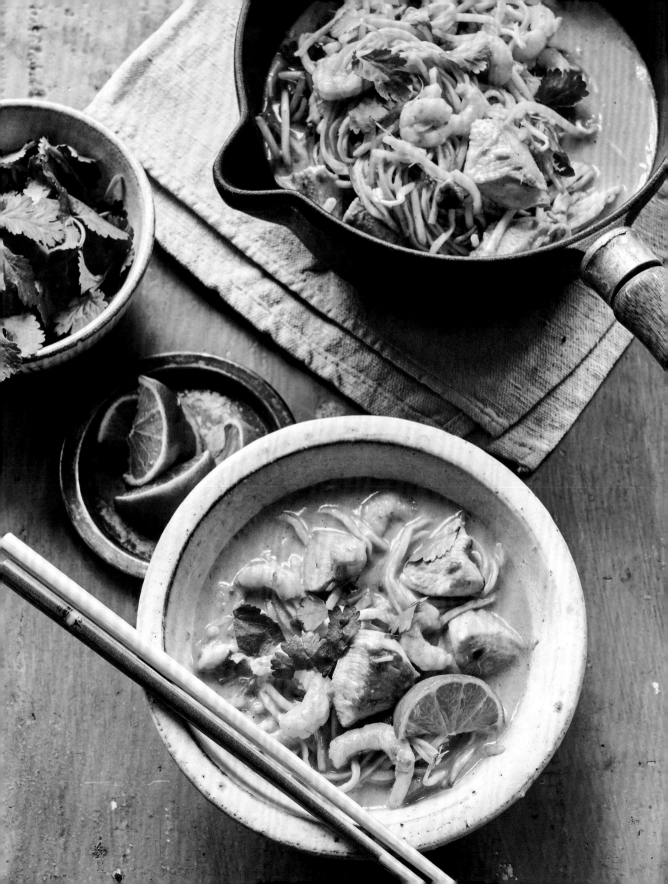

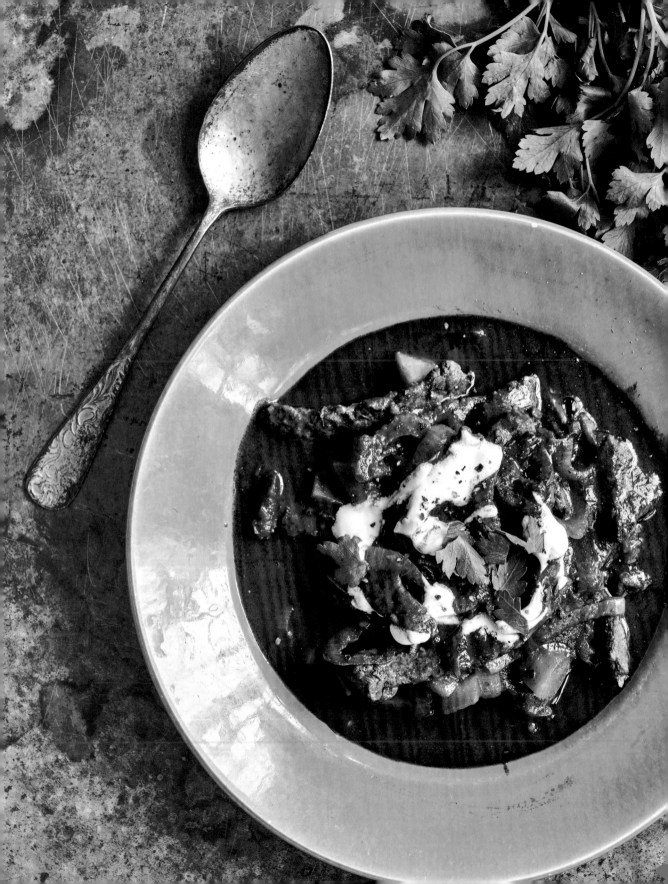

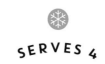

BEEF GOULASH SOUP

Based on traditional Hungarian goulash, this is a warming, hearty and filling soup that will serve as a main meal. The flavours work well for kids, too, as it's not spicy, just full of flavour. If I'm serving this to my children, I blend their portions into a smoother soup so they don't get fussy about 'bits' and they happily eat it.

CALORIES PER SERVING: 259
PREP TIME: 15 MINUTES
COOK TIME: 1¾ HOURS

spray oil
3 onions, sliced
2 celery sticks, sliced
400g (14oz) thin-cut lean beef
   steaks, cut into fine strips
1 teaspoon caraway seeds
3 garlic cloves, crushed
1 red chilli, deseeded and finely
   chopped
400g (14oz) can of chopped
   tomatoes
1.2 litres (2 pints) hot beef stock
2 tablespoons tomato purée
1 tablespoon red wine vinegar
2 carrots, peeled and finely
   chopped
3 tablespoons sweet paprika
salt and pepper

TO SERVE
fat-free Greek yogurt
parsley leaves

1. Preheat the oven to 200°C/180°C fan (400°F), Gas Mark 6.
2. Spray a casserole dish (with a lid) with oil and fry the onions and celery for 10 minutes over a gentle heat, stirring occasionally until the onions are soft and golden. Stir in the beef, caraway seeds, garlic and chilli and stir-fry for 3 minutes.
3. Add the chopped tomatoes, hot stock, tomato purée, vinegar, carrots and paprika, then season and stir.
4. Pop the lid on the pan and place it in the oven for 1½ hours. Remove from the oven and check that the beef is tender and not tough (give it a little longer if it is).
5. Use a hand blender to give a quick blend to the soup, only partly blending it to thicken it up; you don't want to completely purée it.
6. Serve with a dollop of yogurt on top, plenty of parsley and a few grinds of pepper.

NOTE If you want to make this into more of a stew than a soup, use bigger chunks of lean beef (such as lean casserole steak) and add big chunks of sweet potato and sliced red peppers.

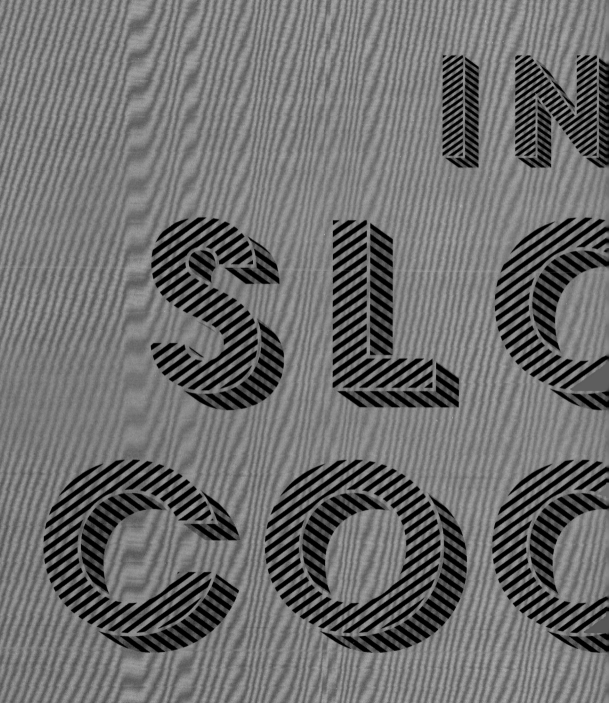

CHAPTER 5

IN
SLO
COD

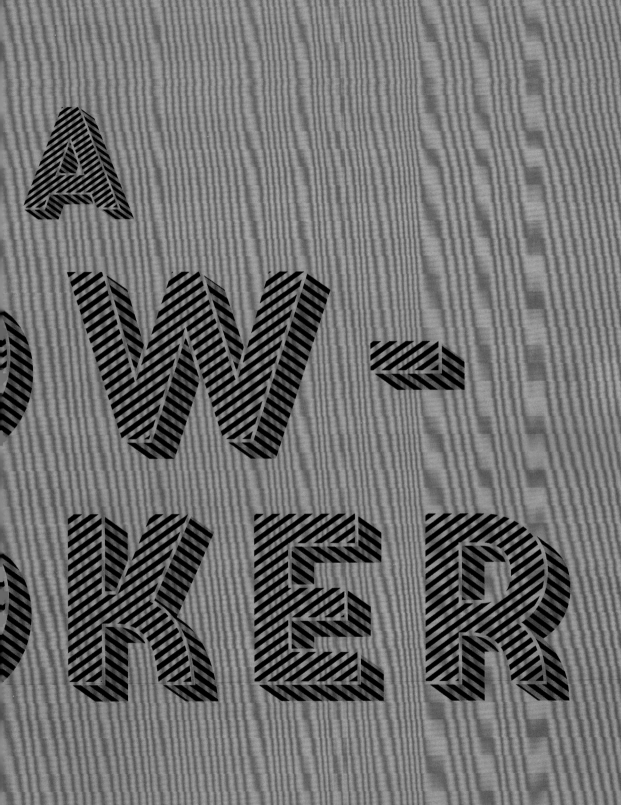

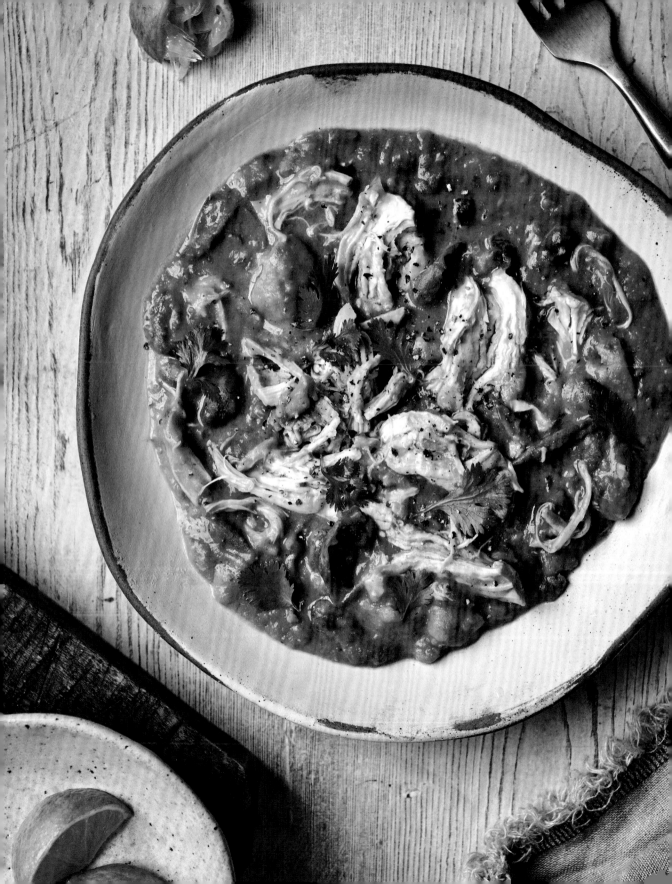

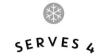

BRAZILIAN-STYLE COCONUT CHICKEN CURRY

This recipe is my 8-year-old's favourite from the whole book. It's creamy from coconut and only very lightly spiced, which means that even for my chilli-averse daughter it is a winner. A hint of peanut butter in the sauce, very tender shredded chicken and pinto beans (great for kids as they are very soft) make this a real family favourite. It's a meal-in-one if you want it to be, or make it go further by serving with rice.

CALORIES PER SERVING: 508
PREP TIME: 10 MINUTES
**COOK TIME: 3 HOURS (HIGH)
OR 5 HOURS (LOW)**

1 onion, finely chopped
2 tablespoons smooth peanut
   butter
finely grated zest and juice of
   1 unwaxed lime, plus lime
   wedges to serve
1 teaspoon chilli flakes
2 garlic cloves, crushed
1 tablespoon ground turmeric
1 tablespoon cornflour
1 chicken stock cube, crumbled
400ml (14fl oz) light coconut
   milk
3 skinless chicken breasts
350g (12oz) sweet potatoes,
   peeled and chopped
400g (14oz) can of pinto beans,
   drained and rinsed
250g (9oz) cherry tomatoes,
   halved
salt and pepper
coriander leaves, to serve

1. Put the onion into the slow-cooker pot with the peanut butter, lime zest and juice, chilli flakes, crushed garlic, turmeric, cornflour, crumbled stock cube and coconut milk and stir everything together thoroughly.
2. Add the whole chicken breasts, sweet potatoes, pinto beans and tomatoes, season well and stir again, place the lid on and cook on high for 3 hours or on low for 5 hours.
3. When the cooking time is up, use 2 forks to shred the chicken into the sauce. Serve seasoned with pepper, scattered with coriander leaves and with lime wedges on the side.

NOTE To cook this in a regular oven, preheat the oven to 210°C/190°C fan (410°F), Gas Mark 6½. Follow steps 1 and 2, but mix the ingredients in a medium or large casserole dish with a lid. Bake with the lid on for 55 minutes. Check that the chicken is tender and pulls apart easily, then shred the chicken and serve as in step 3.

Want to up the vegetable content in this? Add a few handfuls of chopped spinach at the end of the cooking time, stir it in and leave for a few minutes to wilt into the hot sauce.

CHIPOTLE-SPICED CHICKEN TINGA

A classic Mexican dish. The slow-cooked chicken shreds perfectly into the sauce and I have added black beans to save cooking a separate bean dish. You can find dried chipotle chilli flakes – with a distinctive sweet and smoky flavour – at most big supermarkets, but if you struggle, you may be able to pick up a chipotle paste instead. Serve this over tostadas (tortillas dry-fried in a pan on either side until crisp) with extra toppings such as crunchy shredded lettuce, chopped avocado and tomatoes, jalapeños, and grated cheese, with lime wedges on the side. My Quick Purple Pickle (see page 210) also goes really well with this.

CALORIES PER SERVING: 328
PREP TIME: 5 MINUTES
COOK TIME: 3–4 HOURS (HIGH) OR 6–7 HOURS (LOW)

6 chicken thigh fillets, excess fat trimmed away
1 onion, finely chopped
3 garlic cloves, crushed
400g (14oz) can of black beans, drained and rinsed
3 tablespoons tomato purée
1 tablespoon red wine vinegar
1 tablespoon dried oregano
2 teaspoons chipotle chilli flakes (or see recipe introduction)
1 teaspoon ground cumin
1 teaspoon honey
150ml (¼ pint) chicken stock
salt and pepper

1. Simply place all the ingredients into the slow-cooker pot, season well, mix everything together and cook on high for 3–4 hours, or on low for 6–7 hours.

2. Once the cooking time is up, use 2 forks to thoroughly shred the chicken, mixing it in to absorb the sauce as you go.

NOTE To cook this in a regular oven, preheat the oven to 180°C/160°C fan (350°F), Gas Mark 4. Follow step 1, but double the amount of chicken stock to 300ml (½ pint) and mix the ingredients in a small or medium casserole dish with a lid. Place in the oven and bake with the lid on for 1 hour 20 minutes. Check that the chicken is tender and pulls apart easily, then shred the chicken as in step 2.

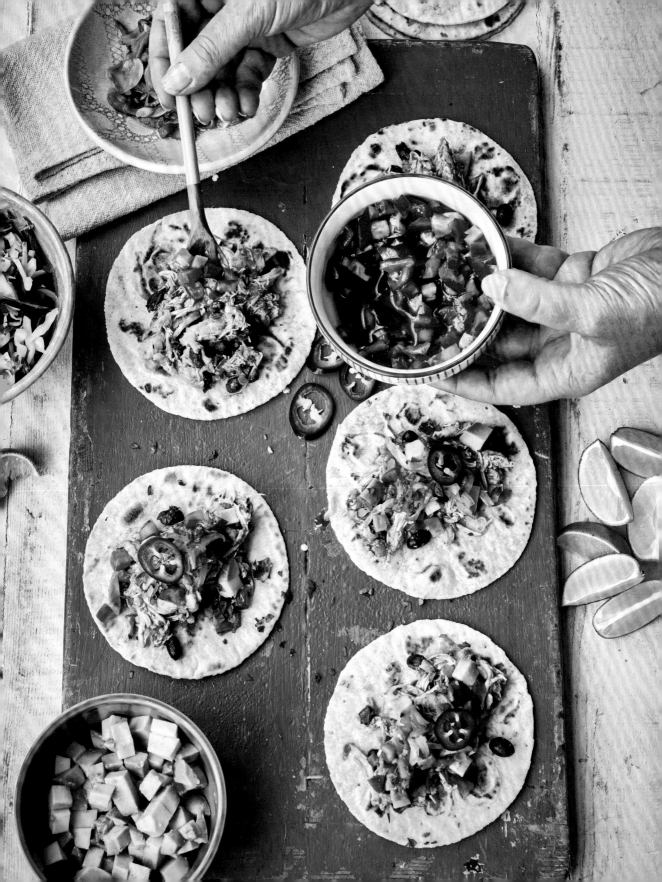

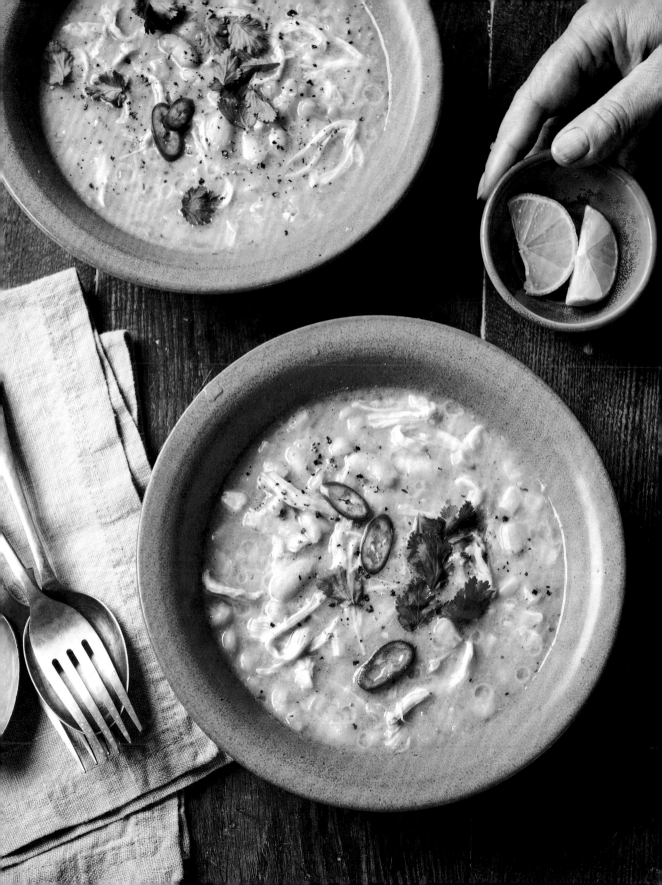

WHITE CHICKEN CHILLI

This is a different take on chilli con carne, where instead of beef and black or kidney beans, I use chicken and cannellini beans. It's a great way to mix up that family favourite. You can serve this with classic accompaniments such as baked potatoes, tortilla chips, guacamole or sliced avocado, grated cheese, jalapeños and lime wedges, or with rice if you want to make it go further.

CALORIES PER SERVING: 447
PREP TIME: 10 MINUTES,
PLUS 5 MINUTES RESTING TIME
COOK TIME: 4–5 HOURS
(HIGH) OR 7–8 HOURS (LOW)

600g (1lb 5oz) chicken thigh
    fillets (about 6), fat trimmed
    away
1 onion, finely chopped
2 green chillies, deseeded and
    finely chopped
2 × 400g (14oz) cans of cannellini
    beans, drained and rinsed
325g (11½oz) can of sweetcorn,
    drained
2 teaspoons garlic granules
1 teaspoon ground cumin
1 teaspoon dried oregano
500ml (18fl oz) chicken stock
3 tablespoons half-fat crème
    fraîche
1 tablespoon cornflour
salt and pepper

TO SERVE
coriander leaves
sliced green chillies
lime wedges

1. Place the chicken, onion, chillies, cannellini beans, sweetcorn, garlic granules, cumin, oregano and chicken stock into the slow-cooker pot and season with salt and pepper.
2. Give everything a mix, pop the lid on and cook on high for 4–5 hours, or on low for 7–8 hours.
3. Towards the end of the cooking time, in a small bowl, combine the crème fraîche and cornflour.
4. Use 2 forks to shred the chicken thighs in the slow-cooker bowl, then stir in the crème fraîche mixture. Leave for 5 minutes, then stir again.
5. Serve with some coriander leaves and sliced green chillies on top and a lime wedge (or see recipe introduction).

NOTE To cook this in a regular oven, preheat the oven to 180°C/160°C fan (350°F), Gas Mark 4. Follow step 1, but mix the ingredients in a medium or large casserole dish with a lid. Place into the oven and cook with the lid on for 1 hour 20 minutes. Follow steps 3 and 4 towards the end of the cooking time and serve as in step 5.

GUACAMOLE
For a simple homemade guacamole to serve 4, mash 2 ripe avocados with a fork and add 1 finely chopped red chilli, the juice of 1 lime, and ½ teaspoon of coarse sea salt. Super-easy, very delicious.

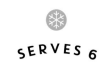

THAI-STYLE PUMPKIN SOUP

The slow-cooker takes the pumpkin or squash to perfect tenderness so it blends perfectly into a velvety soup. Please be aware that different Thai curry pastes have different levels of heat, so do have a look at the instructions on the one you buy to note the recommended amount to use.

CALORIES PER SERVING: 179
PREP TIME: 20 MINUTES
COOK TIME: 4 HOURS (HIGH)
OR 6 HOURS (LOW)

1.5kg (3lb 5oz) pumpkin or butternut squash, peeled, deseeded and cut into large chunks
1 carrot, peeled and sliced
1 onion, finely chopped
400ml (14fl oz) can of light coconut milk
1 litre (1¾ pints) hot chicken stock
1 tablespoon Thai red curry paste (see recipe introduction)
1 teaspoon salt
1 teaspoon honey
2 teaspoons fish sauce
juice of 1 lime

TO SERVE
coriander leaves
sliced red chillies
pepper

1. Put the pumpkin or squash, carrot, onion and coconut milk into the slow-cooker pot.
2. Make up the hot stock in a jug and stir in the red curry paste to dissolve. Pour it into the slow-cooker pot.
3. Add the salt, stir, place the lid on the slow-cooker and cook on high for 4 hours, or on low for 6 hours.
4. Once cooked and the pumpkin or squash is tender, use a hand blender to whizz it into a creamy soup, then stir in the honey, fish sauce and lime juice and season with pepper. Serve with coriander leaves and sliced red chillies.

NOTE To cook this in a regular oven, preheat the oven to 200°C/180°C fan (400°F), Gas Mark 6. Follow steps 1–3, but mix the ingredients in a large casserole dish with a lid and cook in the oven with the lid on for 45 minutes. Check that the squash is tender, then blend the soup with a hand blender and add the remaining ingredients as in step 4.

HOW TO PREPARE BUTTERNUT SQUASH
Start by cutting 5mm (¼ inch) off both the top and bottom of the squash using a large, sharp knife. Use a sharp Y-shaped vegetable peeler to peel off the outer layer. Stand the squash upright and make one long cut down the middle, from top to the bottom, to cut it in half. Use a metal spoon to scrape out the seeds and stringy pulp from the cavity, then cut the halves into slices or cubes, as desired

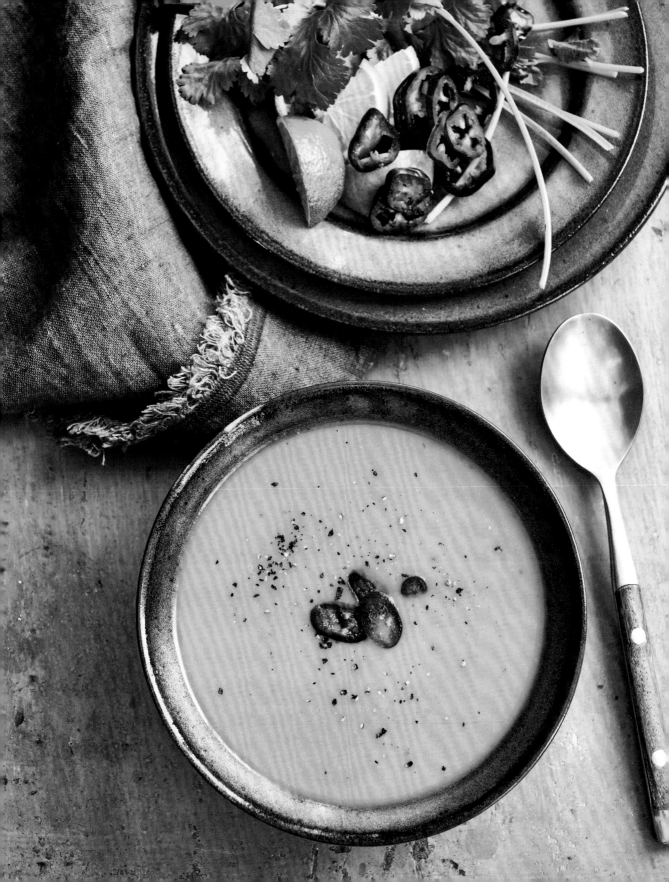

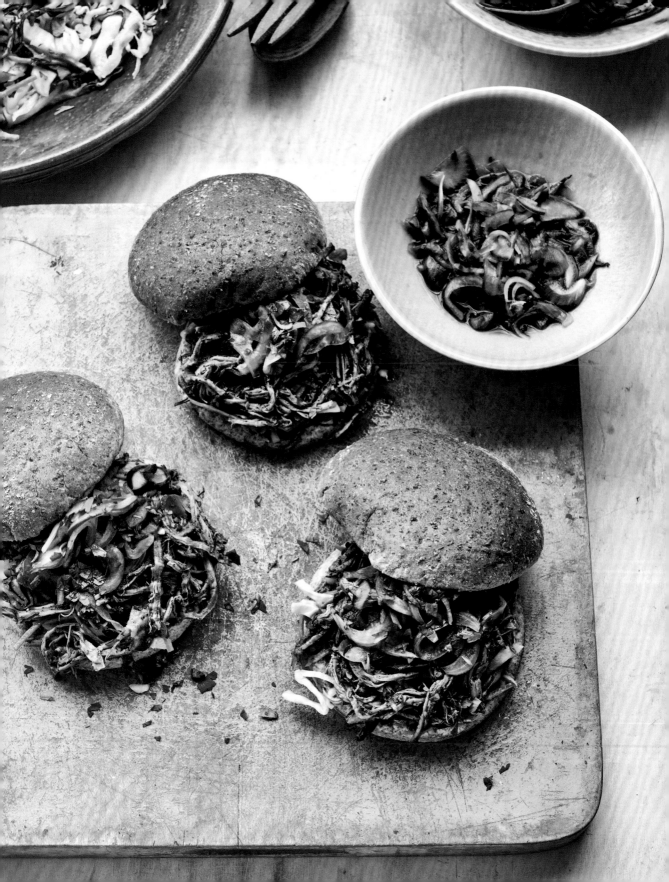

COFFEE-RUBBED BARBECUE PULLED PORK

The slow-cooker really is a hero when it comes to pulled pork, I've never had a batch that wasn't perfectly tender and delicious. Serve this with lightly toasted wholemeal baps, Super Slaw and Quick Purple Pickle (see pages 183 and 210), or simply cut carrots into matchsticks and finely shred cabbage to go in the baps and scatter over some fresh coriander.

CALORIES PER SERVING: 274
PREP TIME: 10 MINUTES
COOK TIME: 4–6 HOURS (HIGH) OR 6–8 HOURS (LOW)

2 × pork tenderloins (total weight about 1kg/2lb 4oz)

FOR THE SPICE MIX
2 teaspoons smoked paprika
1 tablespoon fine-ground espresso coffee
1 teaspoon garlic granules
1 teaspoon coarse sea salt
½ teaspoon cayenne pepper

FOR THE SAUCE
150ml (¼ pint) chicken stock
2 tablespoons balsamic vinegar
2 tablespoons tomato purée
1 tablespoon honey
1 tablespoon Worcestershire sauce

1. Make up the spice rub by mixing everything in a bowl.
2. Place the pork tenderloins into the slow-cooker pot and rub them all over with the spice mix.
3. Make up the sauce by mixing all the ingredients together in a small bowl. Pour this around the pork, then place the lid on the slow-cooker. Cook on low for 6–8 hours (this will give the best results), or on high for 4–6 hours.
4. Use 2 forks to shred the tender pork and mix it into the juices to absorb the flavours.

NOTE To cook this in a regular oven, preheat the oven to 180°C/160°C fan (350°F), Gas Mark 4. Follow steps 1 and 2, but mix the ingredients in a medium casserole dish with a lid. Bake with the lid on for 2 hours.

WHAT TO DO WITH LEFTOVERS
If I have leftover pulled pork, I often use it to make burritos. I have a very specific way that I like to layer them up which I think makes them perfect. Buy large tortillas and spread 1 tablespoon of refried beans over the middle of each. Next add the (reheated) pulled pork, then grated cheese, salsa, jalapeños and shredded Little Gem lettuce and finally squeeze over lime juice. Sometimes I also add extra whole beans such as canned pinto beans or black beans. See page 103 for how to roll a burrito.

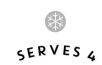

PORK AFRITADA

Afritada is a stew that originated in the Philippines, made from chicken, beef or pork in a tomato-based sauce with potatoes and carrots. The kids loved this version with added hotdog sausages, they add great smoky flavour and are always a popular addition! Pork in the slow-cooker is always a winner and pork tenderloins are a great lean cut but still cook to fall-apart tenderness. This is great bowl food; there is no need for side dishes, but if you want it to go further you can serve it with rice.

CALORIES PER SERVING: 482
PREP TIME: 20 MINUTES
COOK TIME: 5–6 HOURS
(HIGH) OR 7–8 HOURS (LOW)

500g (1lb 2oz) pork tenderloin, sliced
2 large potatoes (total weight 400g/14oz), peeled and cut into large chunks
16 Chantenay (baby) carrots, tops cut off and peeled
1 onion, finely chopped
3 garlic cloves, crushed
150g (5½oz) frozen peas
4 hotdog sausages or frankfurters, sliced
6 salad tomatoes (total weight 350–400g/13–14oz), chopped
200ml (7fl oz) chicken stock
3 tablespoons light soy sauce
2 tablespoons tomato purée
½ tablespoon fish sauce
1 teaspoon honey
2 bay leaves
salt and pepper

1. Add all the ingredients to the slow-cooker pot, season well and stir thoroughly.
2. Cook on high for 5–6 hours, or on low for 7–8 hours. The pork should be tender and easy to pull apart. If it is still tough, you need to cook it for longer.
3. Remove the bay leaves before serving.

NOTE To cook this in a regular oven, preheat the oven to 190°C/170°C fan (375°F), Gas Mark 5. Follow step 1, but increase the amount of chicken stock to 500ml (18fl oz) and mix the ingredients in a medium or large casserole dish with a lid. Place in the oven and bake with the lid on for 1½ hours.

To cook this with chicken, use chicken thigh fillets and reduce the cooking time to 3–4 hours on high, or 6–7 hours on low. For beef, use lean diced beef and keep the cooking times the same as the pork.

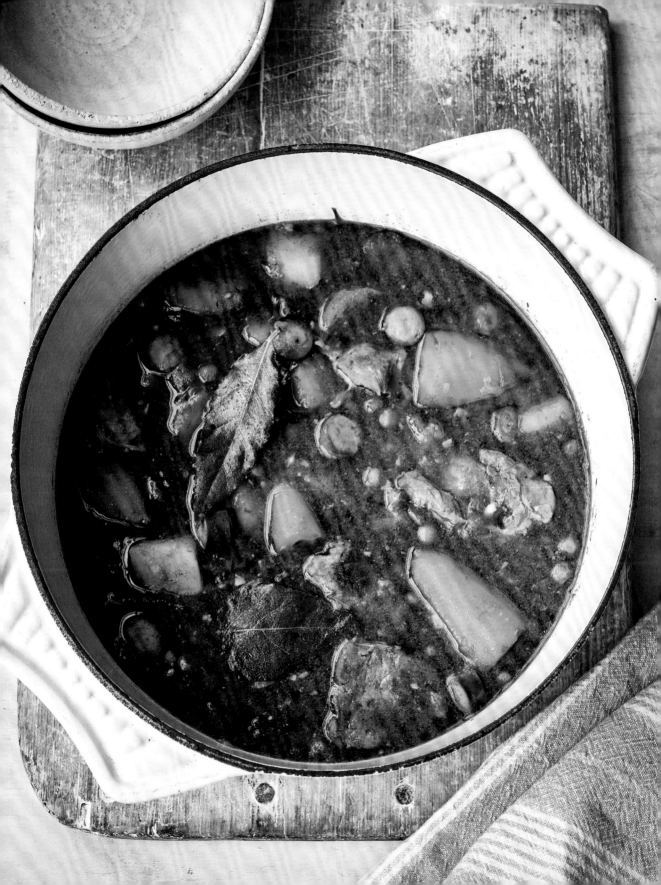

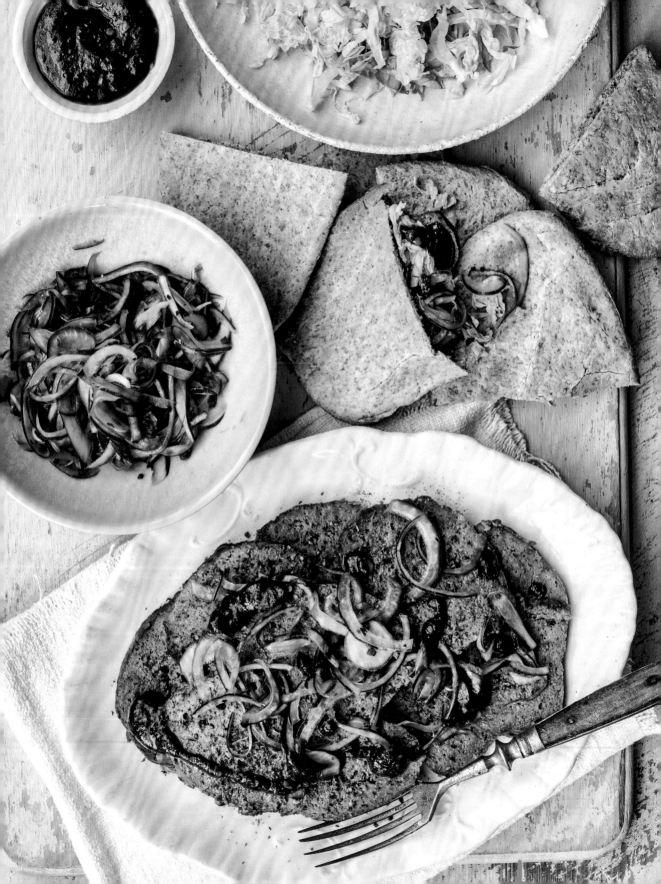

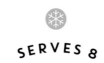

FAKEAWAY DONER KEBAB

This is such an easy family-friendly recipe to put together. I use a mix of minced beef and lamb, but you can use one or the other if you prefer. A warning: this is not pretty, but it's so tasty that you will forget all about its looks! Try it with Super Slaw and Quick Purple Pickle (see pages 183 and 210), warm pitta breads (for homemade see page 202) and chilli sauce.

CALORIES PER SERVING: 195
PREP TIME: 5 MINUTES, PLUS COOLING TIME
COOK TIME: 5–6 HOURS ON LOW

500g (1lb 2oz) lean minced beef (less than 5 per cent fat)
500g (1lb 2oz) lean minced lamb (the leanest you can find)
2 teaspoons dried oregano, plus extra to serve
2 teaspoons sweet paprika, plus extra to serve
2 teaspoons ground cumin
2 teaspoons garlic granules
2 teaspoons onion granules
1 teaspoon chilli powder
2 teaspoons salt
1 teaspoon pepper
1 egg

1. Put the meat in a large bowl and use a wooden spoon to mix in the oregano, spices and seasoning. Break up any lumps in the meat, making sure that everything is fully combined. Crack the egg in and mix it into the spiced meat.
2. Using your hands, shape the meat into a large sausage, compressing it as much as possible, and wrap it in foil.
3. Prepare the slow-cooker by scrunching up 2 pieces of foil to place at the bottom of the pot.
4. Use a sharp knife to poke a few holes in the underside of the foil containing the meat, to allow some of the fat to escape during cooking. Place the kebab on top of the scrunched foil in the slow-cooker pot (or cut the sausage in half, wrap the two halves in foil and place them side by side to fit.)
5. Place the lid on and cook on low for 5–6 hours.
6. Remove the meat from the foil, scrape away any residue sitting on the surface of the meat and sprinkle with paprika and oregano. Allow to cool slightly, then slice as finely as you can with a sharp knife.

NOTE To cook this in a regular oven, preheat the oven to 170°C/150°C fan (340°F), Gas Mark 3½. Follow steps 1 and 2, place the foil-wrapped kebab on a baking tray, and bake for 1½ hours. Open the foil to expose the kebab, increase the oven temperature to 220°C/200°C fan (425°F), Gas Mark 7 and cook for a further 10 minutes to brown. Once cooked, remove the kebab (discard any liquid) and place it on a plate to rest for a few minutes before sprinkling with paprika and oregano and slicing as in step 6.

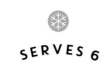

CASUAL LASAGNE

I love lasagne, but it's one of those dishes that often takes just a little more effort than I'm willing to put in. This method is a bit of a game-changer. Of course it is different from the carefully prepared, oven-baked counterpart: it's not in neat and tidy layers, but messy, comforting and full of flavour! It's just so quick and easy to put together that it's a total slow-cooker winner. You may feel sceptical about not pre-cooking the mince, but there is no need in this version, the meat will still be tender and perfect. I serve this up with a big salad on the side.

CALORIES PER SERVING: 422
PREP TIME: 5 MINUTES
COOK TIME: 4–5 HOURS ON LOW

500g (1lb 2oz) lean minced beef (less than 5 per cent fat)
400g (14oz) can of chopped tomatoes
500ml (18fl oz) tomato passata
2 tablespoons tomato purée
1 tablespoon balsamic vinegar
2 carrots, peeled and grated
2 teaspoons garlic granules
2 teaspoons onion granules
1 teaspoon sweet paprika
1 tablespoon dried oregano, plus extra for sprinkling
1 beef stock cube
6 lasagne sheets
300g (10½oz) fat-free cottage cheese
105g (3¾oz) Cheddar cheese, grated
125g (4½oz) mozzarella cheese, torn
salt and pepper
curly parsley leaves, to serve

1. In a large bowl, mix the minced beef, chopped tomatoes, passata, tomato purée, balsamic vinegar, carrots, garlic granules, onion granules, paprika and oregano together, breaking up the minced beef so there are no large chunks and it's well combined with the sauce. Crush the beef stock cube and sprinkle in, and season with salt and pepper before stirring again.

2. Spoon one-third of the meat mixture into the slow-cooker pot, then cover with 2 lasagne sheets (break these up to fit them to your pot). Spread over one-third of the cottage cheese to cover the lasagne sheets and one-third of the Cheddar. Repeat this twice more so you have 3 layers. On the top layer, break up the mozzarella to cover and sprinkle over a little extra oregano.

3. Turn the slow-cooker to low, and cook for 4–5 hours. If you would like the cheese to be browned on top before serving, just pop the pot under a hot grill for a few minutes.

4. Serve scattered with curly parsley.

NOTE To cook this in a regular oven, preheat the oven to 170°C/150°C fan (340°F), Gas Mark 3½. Follow steps 1 and 2, but layer the lasagne in a medium or large casserole dish with a lid. Bake with the lid on for 2 hours. Serve as in step 4.

I recommend sticking to the low setting for this one to be perfect, as it doesn't work so well on high.

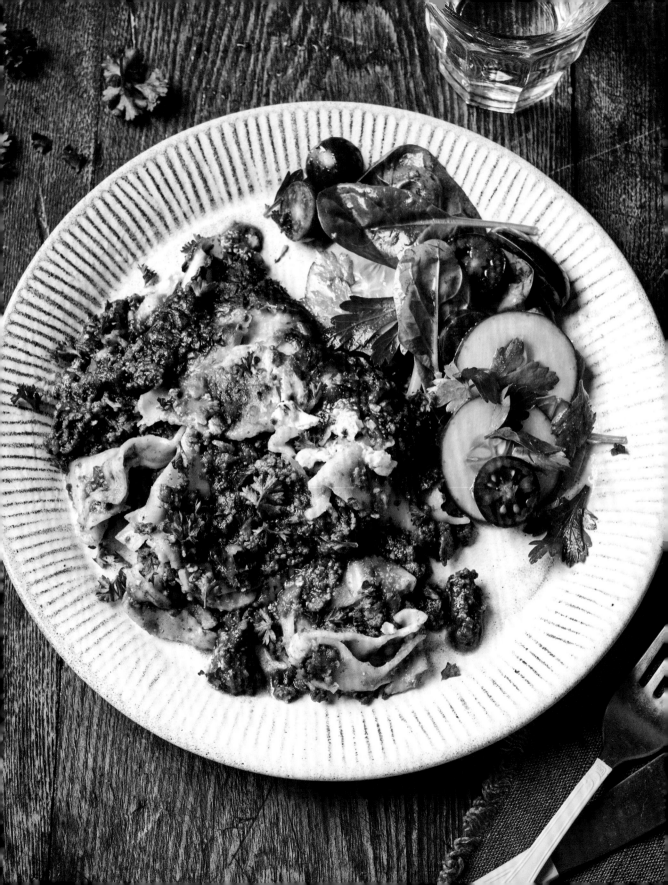

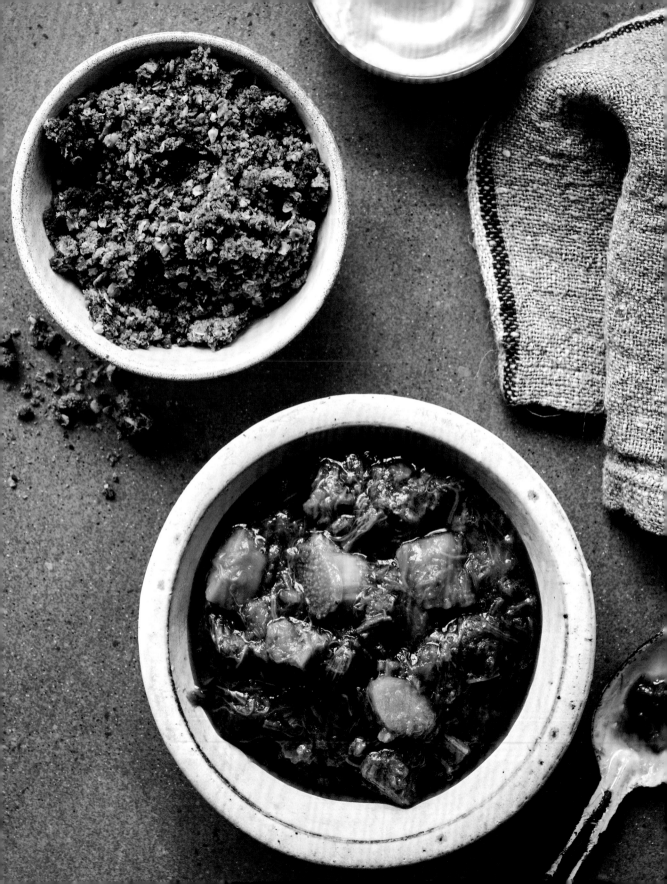

RHUBARB, STRAWBERRY & APPLE COMPOTE

A sweet and delicious combination of fruit that is perfect to serve over porridge or yogurt for breakfast, or with hot custard or a crumble mix for dessert. Slow-cooking this means that there's no pan-watching or risk of it burning, and it tenderizes the fruit beautifully. I use frozen strawberries for this as, once thawed, they are already softened and will be as tender as the rest of the fruit.

CALORIES PER SERVING: 79
PREP TIME: 5 MINUTES
COOK TIME: 1.5 HOURS (HIGH) OR 3 HOURS (LOW)

400g (14oz) rhubarb, washed, trimmed and cut into 1cm (½ inch) pieces

2 large cooking apples (total weight about 400g/14oz), peeled, cored and chopped

150g (5½oz) frozen strawberries

50g (1¾oz) caster sugar

2 teaspoons vanilla extract

1. Place the rhubarb, apples and strawberries into the slow-cooker pot and add the sugar and vanilla.
2. Mix everything together, place the lid on and cook on high for 1½ hours, or on low for 3 hours.
3. When cooked, the fruit should be tender. Use a wooden spoon to break up and blend it all together. You can serve this hot or cold.

NOTE To cook this in a regular oven, preheat the oven to 200°C/180°C fan (400°F), Gas Mark 6. Follow steps 1 and 2, but mix the ingredients in a medium-sized casserole dish with a lid. Bake in the oven with the lid on for 35 minutes, stirring after the first 15 minutes to coat everything in the juices at the bottom of the pan. When the cooking time has ended, the fruit should all be tender and easily broken up with a wooden spoon.

NOTE To make a change, add ½ teaspoon of ground cinnamon to the mix instead of the vanilla extract.

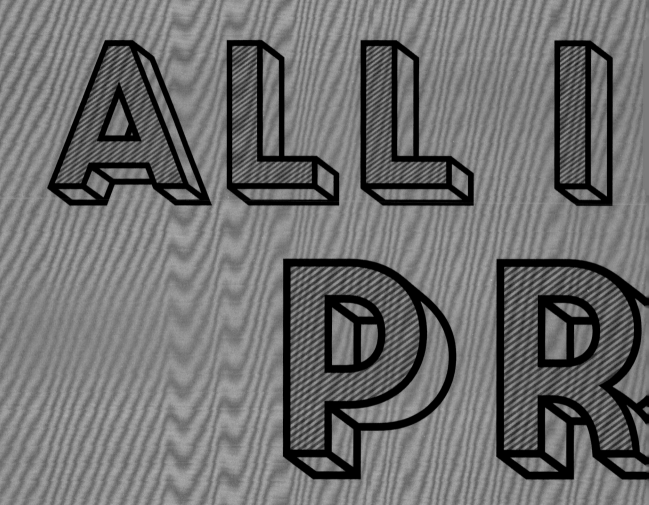

CHAPTER 6

ALL I
PR

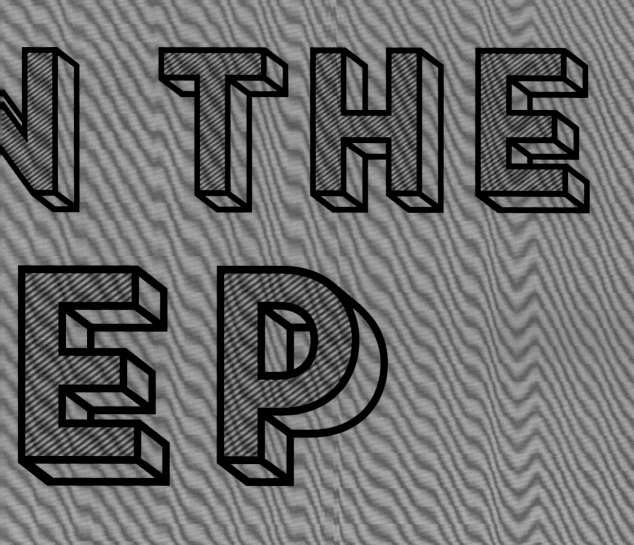

SERVES 2

WARM BURST TOMATO, ROCKET & MOZZARELLA

I love the classic combination of tomato, rocket and mozzarella, but roasting the tomatoes first with garlic takes it to the next level. I happily eat this as a stand-alone dish, but it also makes a great side salad. Try adding 1 tablespoon of my savoury Crunchy Seed Sprinkle (see page 218) for extra crunch. If you want to bulk this up, add a pre-cooked grain mix such as quinoa and bulgur wheat.

CALORIES PER SERVING: 228
PREP TIME: 5 MINUTES, PLUS
COOLING TIME
COOK TIME: 20 MINUTES

250g (9oz) red and yellow cherry
    tomatoes, halved
2 garlic cloves, crushed
1 teaspoon olive oil
60g (2¼oz) rocket, roughly
    chopped
125g (4½oz) mozzarella pearls,
    or just mozzarella torn into
    small pieces
½ tablespoon balsamic vinegar
coarse sea salt and pepper
torn basil leaves, to serve

1. Preheat the oven to 240°C/220°C fan (475°F), Gas Mark 9.
2. In a medium-sized bowl, mix together the tomatoes, garlic and olive oil, then spread this mixture into a single layer on a baking tray. Season with salt and pepper.
3. Roast the tomatoes for 20 minutes (keep a bit of an eye on them to make sure they don't burn). Remove them from the oven and allow to cool slightly.
4. Toss the tomatoes in a serving bowl with the rocket and mozzarella, drizzle over the balsamic vinegar, then finish with torn basil leaves and a small grinding of coarse sea salt.

THE BALSAMIC BOOST

Balsamic vinegar is such a useful and powerful ingredient. I use it for roasting vegetables, in salad dressings, in tomato sauces and casseroles. You can pick up great-value balsamic vinegar for day-to-day use, but consider a more expensive bottle for dressing salads such as this. Often the more expensive balsamic vinegars will have a thicker consistency which coats salad leaves rather than just dripping to the bottom of the bowl, plus the flavour is far more developed. A bottle of nice balsamic vinegar can last for years and will go really far.

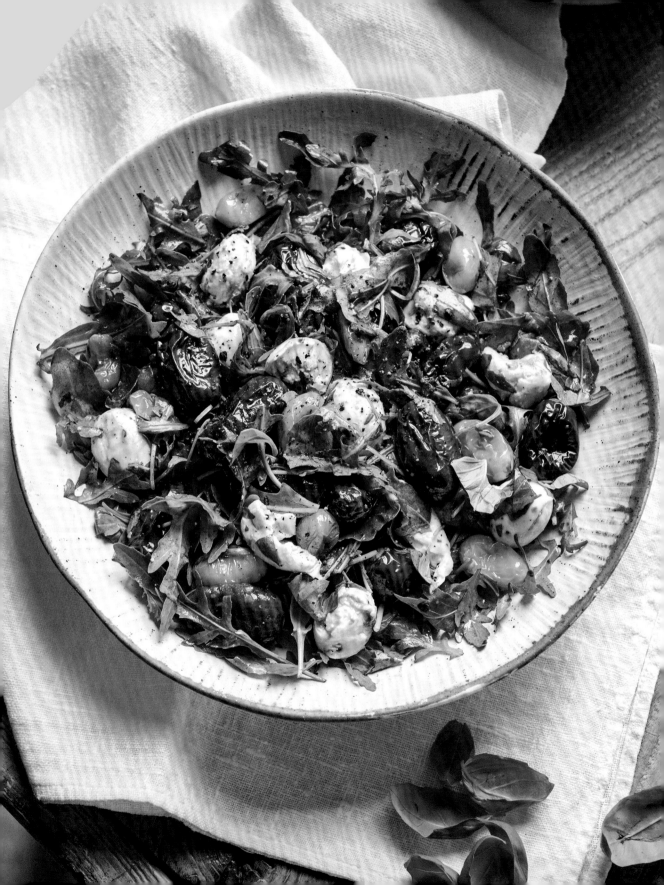

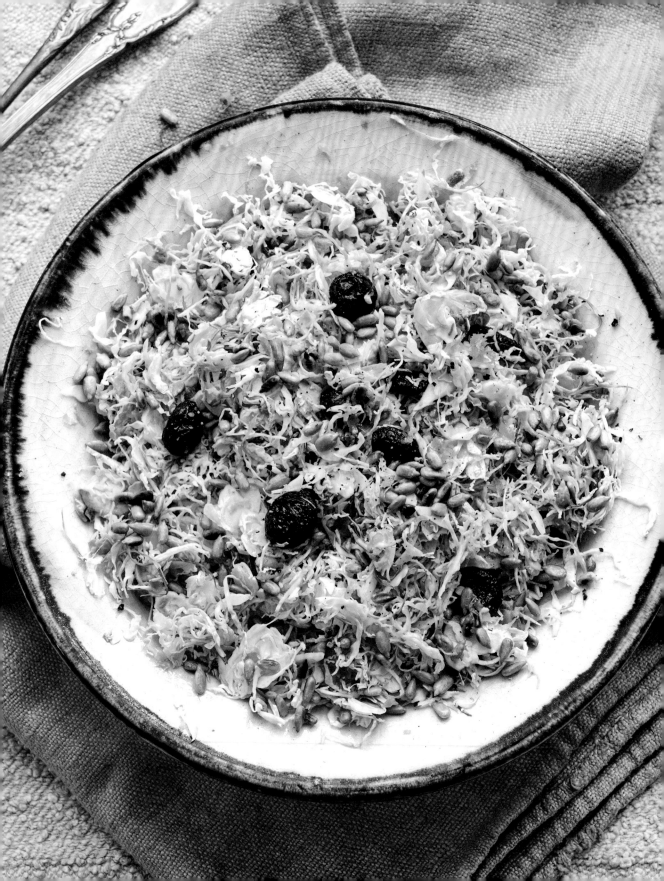

EVERY DAY IS CHRISTMAS SALAD

Shredded Brussels sprouts, dried cranberries and a zesty honey-orange dressing take some traditional Christmas ingredients and turn them into a delicious and surprisingly summery salad. Depending on where you live, Brussels sprouts are often available year-round; I love their crunch and the sweet nutty taste of them in a salad. This makes a great side dish to go with a barbecue in the summer, and it's also a perfect way to use up great-value Brussels sprouts in the winter months. Try it alongside cold cuts, quiche or my Coffee-Rubbed Barbecue Pulled Pork (see page 165).

CALORIES PER SERVING: 90
PREP TIME: 20 MINUTES
COOK TIME: 2 MINUTES

450g (1lb) Brussels sprouts, prepared and finely shredded (see box below)
25g (1oz) dried cranberries
2 tablespoons sunflower seeds

FOR THE DRESSING
finely grated zest of 1 unwaxed orange
1 tablespoon apple cider vinegar
1 teaspoon honey
salt and pepper

1. Prepare and shred the sprouts (see box below).
2. Make up the dressing in a small bowl by stirring all the ingredients vigorously until the honey has dissolved.
3. In a serving bowl, toss together the shredded sprouts and dried cranberries.
4. Lightly toast the sunflower seeds by dry-frying them in a small frying pan over a high heat for 1–2 minutes.
5. Add the sunflower seeds to the sprouts and cranberries, pour over the dressing, toss everything together and serve.

HOW TO PREPARE BRUSSELS SPROUTS
Rinse the sprouts in a colander under running water, then pull away and discard any loose, damaged or yellowed leaves. Trim away the discoloured base with a sharp knife. To shred them, cut the sprout in half lengthways, then finely slice the halves.

TEX-MEX MACARONI SALAD

A super-quick pasta salad to rustle up that requires very little chopping. With a light Tex-Mex style dressing, this salad is also really versatile as a side dish. I make it as a pot-luck for friends' barbecues, to go with fajita-seasoned chicken or pulled pork. You can customize this to your own tastes and to what ingredients you have available or in season. Try substituting the black beans for pinto beans, use different shapes of pasta (though larger varieties need to cook for longer), or add extra vegetables such as avocado, red onion, green beans, carrots and baby tomatoes. You can also change the level of spiciness by adjusting the amount of jalapeños.

CALORIES PER SERVING: 331
PREP TIME: 10 MINUTES
COOK TIME: 10 MINUTES

250g (9oz) macaroni
400g (14oz) can of black beans, drained and rinsed
150g (5½oz) frozen sweetcorn, defrosted
1 red pepper, deseeded and finely chopped
4 spring onions, sliced
large handful of coriander leaves, finely chopped
salt and pepper

FOR THE DRESSING
2 tablespoons fat-free Greek yogurt
1 garlic clove, crushed
½ teaspoon smoked paprika
2 tablespoons finely chopped jalapeños
juice of 1 lime
pepper

1. Bring a large pan of water to the boil and add 2 teaspoons of salt. Pour in the macaroni and simmer fast for 5 minutes.
2. Add the black beans and sweetcorn and simmer for another 5 minutes, or until the pasta is cooked.
3. Drain the pasta, beans and sweetcorn and give it a quick rinse under cold water. Drain very well. Place in a serving bowl and stir in the pepper, spring onions and coriander.
4. Make up the dressing in a small bowl by stirring all the ingredients vigorously. Add it to the salad, season well, then stir to combine everything.
5. Serve warm or cold.

NOTE This is an easy salad to customize: make it Greek-style by replacing the smoked paprika, jalapeños and lime with my Greek Seasoning Blend (see page 222) and replacing the beans and sweetcorn with baby tomatoes and cucumber. Or make it a tandoori pasta salad by combining the Greek fat-free yogurt with 1 teaspoon of my Tandoori Spice Blend (see page 222), 1 crushed garlic clove and the juice of 1 lemon, adding grated carrot, chopped tomatoes and chickpeas.

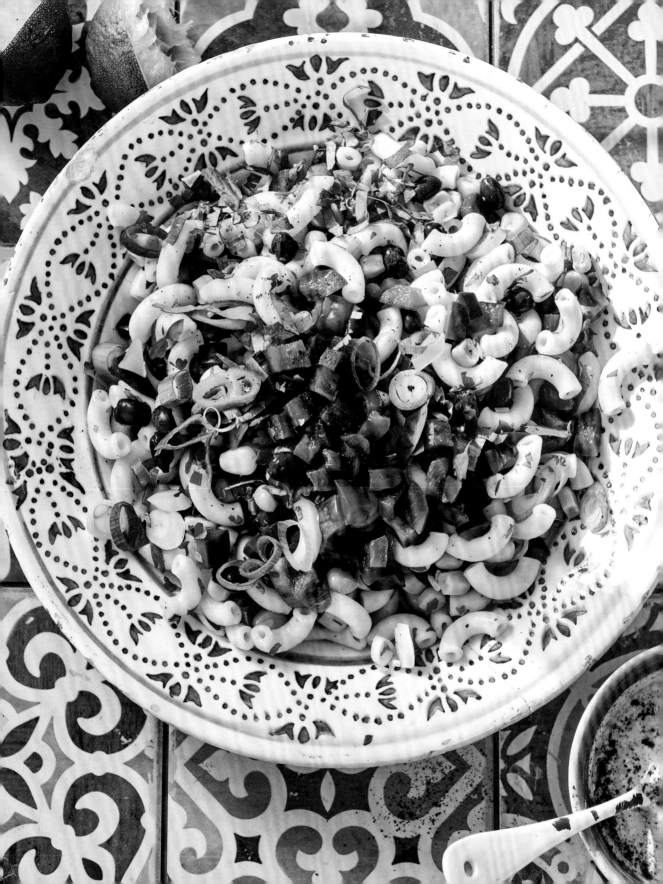

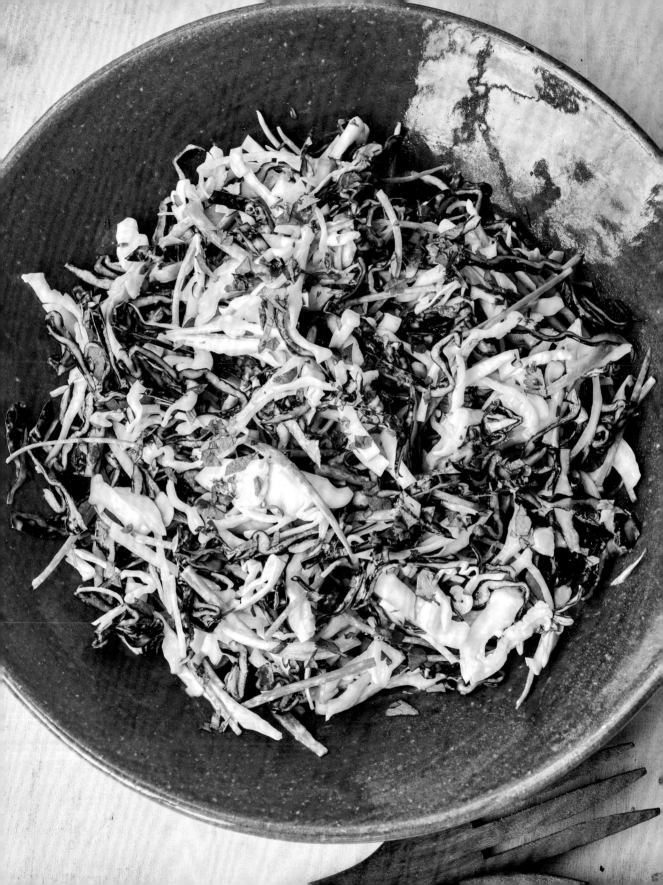

SUPER SLAW

I used to think that I hated coleslaw, but it turns out that I just couldn't stomach that sloppy, mayonnaise-covered version. As soon as I started making my own, it was a complete game-changer. Fat-free Greek yogurt makes a great light alternative to mayonnaise. This coleslaw is a perfect accompaniment to my Fakeaway Doner Kebab and Quick Purple Pickle, but also makes a brilliant side dish to Coffee-Rubbed Barbecue Pulled Pork (see pages 169, 210 and 165). It's beautiful in a burger or hotdog, or served with grilled halloumi.

CALORIES PER SERVING: 67
PREP TIME: 10 MINUTES
COOK TIME: NONE

½ small red cabbage
½ small green cabbage
2 large carrots
100g (3½oz) fat-free Greek
   yogurt
1 tablespoon honey
1 teaspoon Dijon mustard
1 garlic clove, crushed
juice of 1 lemon
salt
handful of herbs, such as
   parsley, mint or coriander,
   to serve

1. To prepare the cabbage, remove the bruised outer leaves, cut it into quarters, cut out the core, then finely slice into shreds.
2. Pop the shredded cabbage in a large bowl and grate in the carrots.
3. Mix up the yogurt, honey, mustard, garlic, lemon juice and a large pinch of salt in a small bowl. Dress the coleslaw with this only once you are ready to serve it.
4. Scatter with whatever herbs you have.

NOTE You can spice this up with chopped chilli, or add some flavours to complement a particular dish: for example, to go alongside an Indian meal, swap out the Dijon mustard for ½ teaspoon of ground turmeric and swap the honey for mango chutney, then scatter with cumin seeds to serve.

> **RAVISHING ROAST CABBAGE**
> This makes a lovely side dish to a roast dinner, or to sausages and grilled meats. To roast cabbage, preheat the oven to 220°C/200°C fan (425°F), Gas Mark 7. Shred the cabbage and mix it in an oven tray with 2 sliced onions, 2 tablespoons apple cider vinegar, salt and pepper and some spray oil. Roast it for 15 minutes, give it a stir, then roast it for another 20 minutes.

LIGHT NEW POTATO & GREEN BEAN SALAD

A light and summery salad that's perfect alongside grilled meat or fish, or cold cuts. You can eat it warm or cold.

CALORIES PER SERVING: 207
PREP TIME: 10 MINUTES
COOK TIME: 20 MINUTES

1kg (2lb 4oz) new potatoes, cut into roughly uniform bite-sized pieces
200g (7oz) green beans, trimmed
4 spring onions, finely sliced
1 tablespoon chopped parsley leaves
½ tablespoon chopped tarragon leaves

FOR THE DRESSING
3 tablespoons apple cider vinegar
2 garlic cloves, crushed
1 teaspoon Dijon mustard
½ teaspoon honey
½ teaspoon olive oil
salt and pepper

1. In a medium-sized saucepan of boiling water, simmer the potatoes for 20 minutes. For the last 2 minutes, add the green beans and simmer them with the potatoes. Scoop the green beans out of the water with a slotted spoon, transfer to a colander and run under cold water to cool them (this keeps them a nice vivid green).
2. Drain the potatoes and allow them to steam while you prepare the dressing.
3. Whisk together the vinegar, garlic, mustard, honey and olive oil in a small bowl and season well.
4. Transfer the potatoes to a serving bowl, add the sliced spring onions and chopped herbs, then pour over the dressing and season with salt and pepper. Add the green beans only when you're ready to serve and stir to coat everything in the dressing.

NOTE You can customize the herbs to your taste. If you aren't fond of tarragon, just leave it out, or replace it with mint. Any quick-cooking seasonal green vegetables can work in the place of green beans, so try asparagus, runner beans or fresh peas. If I'm adding sugarsnap peas, I don't cook them, just add them raw.

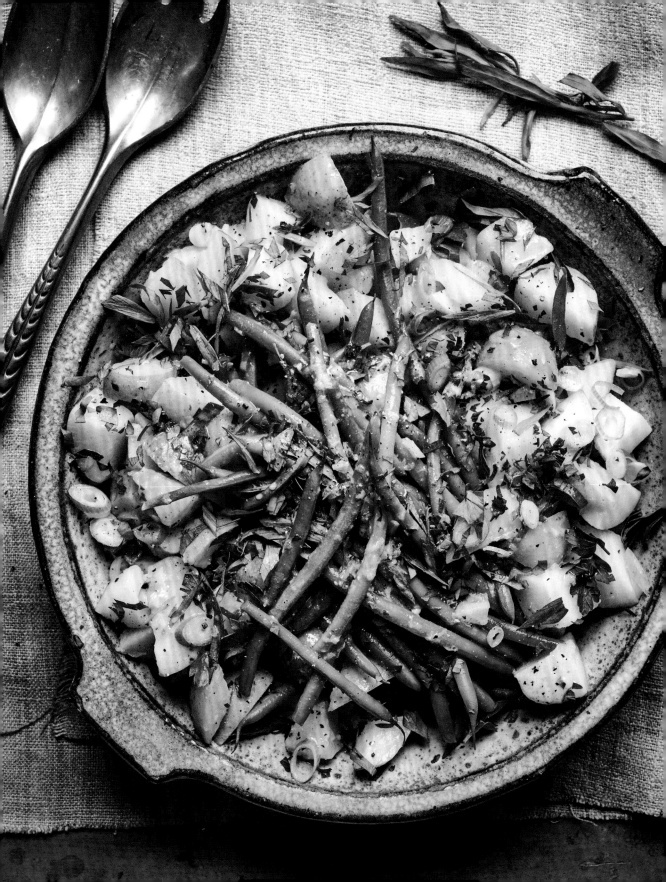

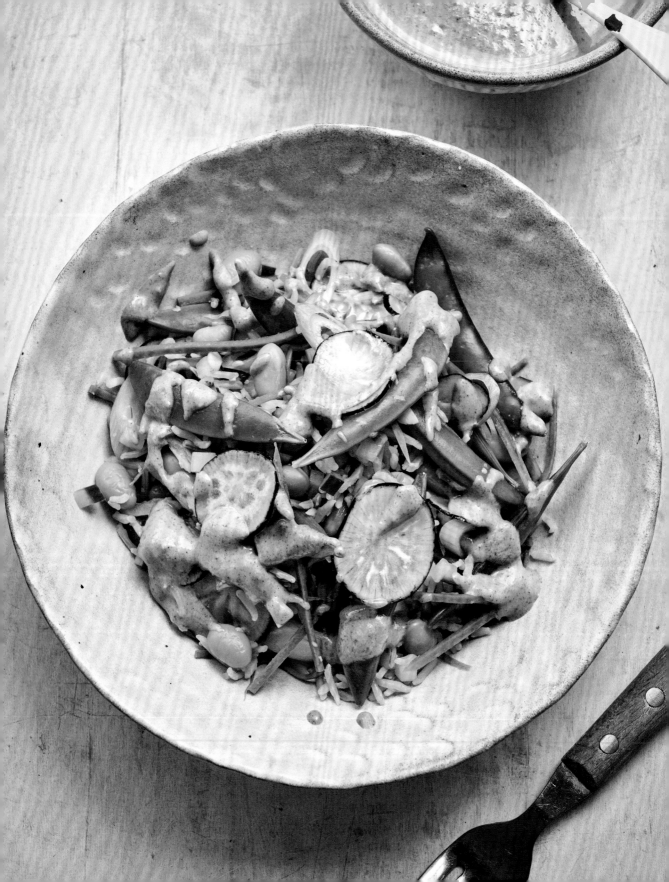

CRUNCHY JAPANESE-STYLE RICE SALAD
WITH YUM-YUM SAUCE

A filling rice salad, with refreshingly crunchy vegetables sharpened with a tasty spicy-sweet dressing. This is ideal for a healthy and filling lunch or dinner and a great dish to bring along to a pot-luck.

CALORIES PER SERVING: 362 (INCLUDING SAUCE)
PREP TIME: 15 MINUTES, PLUS COOLING TIME
COOK TIME: 25 MINUTES, OR AS LONG AS YOUR BROWN RICE TAKES

300g (10½oz) brown rice
150g (5½oz) sugarsnap peas
100g (3½oz) radishes, finely sliced
¼ cucumber, finely chopped
3 spring onions, finely sliced
1 large carrot, peeled and grated
150g (5½oz) edamame beans, podded (defrosted if frozen)
1 quantity Yum-Yum Sauce (see page 221)

1. Cook the brown rice according to the package instructions.
2. While the rice is cooking, prepare the vegetables and the yum-yum sauce.
3. When the rice is cooked, drain it in a sieve, then hold it under running water to cool the rice. Allow it to fully drain by leaving it in the sieve sitting over the still-hot saucepan for a couple of minutes.
4. In a large bowl, mix the cooled brown rice with the sugarsnap peas, radishes, cucumber, spring onions, carrot and edamame.
5. Serve with the yum-yum sauce alongside in a separate bowl, so people can dress their own portion.

NOTE Cooked shredded chicken, prawns, tuna or finely sliced steak go really well with this salad or sauce. It's also a great way to use up crunchy vegetables: try adding peppers, green beans, steamed broccoli or cooked peas and sweetcorn.

SERVES 6

CURRIED BULGUR SALAD

You only need to cook the bulgur wheat here and you can prepare the rest of the ingredients while that is cooking. This delicious vegan salad is full of texture and flavour and can be a meal in itself, or a great side dish. Eat it hot or cold and alter ingredients to suit your own taste.

CALORIES PER SERVING: 261
PREP TIME: 15 MINUTES,
PLUS RESTING TIME
COOK TIME: 12 MINUTES,
OR AS LONG AS YOUR
BULGUR WHEAT TAKES

200g (7oz) bulgur wheat
450ml (16fl oz) vegetable stock
1½ tablespoons mild curry
    powder
3 spring onions, finely sliced
400g (14oz) can of chickpeas,
    drained and rinsed
1 crunchy apple (such as Granny
    Smith or Golden Delicious),
    peeled, cored and finely
    chopped
25g (1oz) raisins
20g (¾oz) flaked almonds
1 large carrot, peeled and grated
1 red pepper, deseeded and finely
    chopped
small handful of mint leaves,
    finely chopped, plus extra
    to serve

FOR THE DRESSING
juice of 1 lemon
1 tablespoon apple cider vinegar
1 tablespoon honey
1 teaspoon coarse sea salt, plus
    extra to taste

1. Put the bulgur wheat into a small- or medium-sized pan, cover with the stock and stir in the curry powder and spring onions. Bring it to a simmer, cover with a lid and allow it to simmer gently for about 12 minutes, or according to the package instructions, until tender.

2. Remove from the heat, fluff it through with a fork, then cover again and leave it to rest for 10 minutes.

3. Transfer the cooked bulgur wheat to a large bowl and add the chickpeas, apple, raisins, almonds, carrot, red pepper and mint.

4. Mix up the dressing ingredients in a small bowl, then pour over the salad, stirring everything together thoroughly to try and coat all the grains and make sure there are no clumps. Season with salt to taste and stir again.

5. Serve scattered with more fresh mint.

NOTE If you are preparing the ingredients while the bulgur wheat is cooking, squeeze some lemon juice over the chopped apple to prevent it from browning while you wait for the bulgur wheat to cook. If you fancy a little bit of heat going through this, add a finely chopped red chilli. If you don't need this to be vegan, then it's a great way to use up leftover roast meat such as chicken, pork, lamb or beef. Simply roughly chop the cold meat and stir it through.

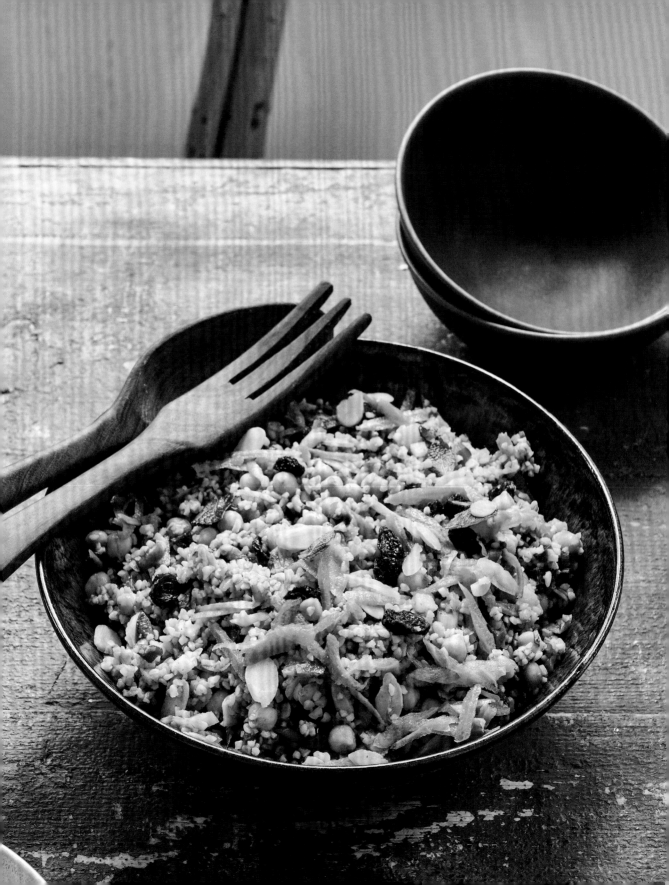

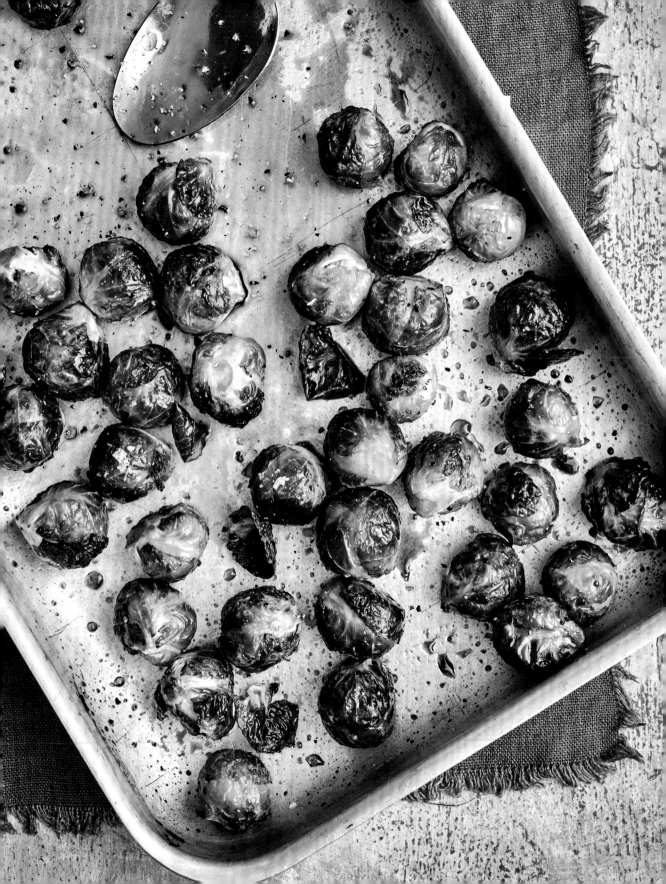

ROAST BRUSSELS SPROUTS

WITH BALSAMIC & HONEY

A dislike of Brussels sprouts can be cured by this very simple way of preparing them. Forget the grey, boiled variety of Christmases past and embrace the sweet and vinegary, slightly charred and crunchy version that this recipe will give you. These make a very versatile side dish for roast dinners, cottage pie, or to sit alongside other salads.

CALORIES PER SERVING: 68
PREP TIME: 15 MINUTES
COOK TIME: 20 MINUTES

450g (1lb) Brussels sprouts, trimmed and halved (see page 179)
spray oil
1 teaspoon honey
1 tablespoon balsamic vinegar
salt and pepper

1. Preheat the oven to 220°C/200°C fan (425°F), Gas Mark 7.
2. Line a baking tray with foil and tip in the sprouts. Spray with oil, season with salt and pepper and roast for 15 minutes.
3. Remove the tray from the oven, stir in the honey and balsamic vinegar to coat all the sprouts and return them back to the oven for 5 more minutes.
4. The sprouts will be golden and slightly charred around the edges. Serve them piping hot.

NOTE You can customize roast sprouts to complement your meal with some of the spice mixes from the Jazz It Up chapter. Try the Tandoori Spice Blend, Greek Seasoning Blend or add my Dukkah Blend for an extra crunch (see pages 222 and 213). Simply replace the balsamic vinegar and honey in step 3 with your chosen spice mix and spray with a little extra oil before roasting for the final 5 minutes.

ROAST CARROT & LENTIL SALAD

WITH FETA & DUKKAH

A hearty warm salad with sweet roasted carrots, earthy lentils, tangy feta cheese and fragrant, toasty dukkah. This is a real hero side dish which complements roast dinners, barbecues or a spread of salads. You can pick up a dukkah mix in most larger supermarkets, but try making your own for incredible flavour (see page 213).

CALORIES PER SERVING: 174
PREP TIME: 10 MINUTES
COOK TIME: 30 MINUTES

500g (1lb 2oz) carrots, peeled and cut into batons
spray oil
400g (14oz) can of green lentils, drained and rinsed
2 roasted red peppers in brine (total weight about 160g/5¾oz), drained and finely sliced
45g (1½oz) feta cheese, chopped small or crumbled
1 tablespoon Dukkah Blend (for homemade, see page 213)

1. Preheat the oven to 200°C/180°C fan (400°F), Gas Mark 6.
2. Place the carrots in a roasting pan, spray with oil and roast for 25 minutes.
3. Stir the lentils and peppers into the carrots, crumble the feta over the top, then sprinkle over the dukkah.
4. Return to the oven and roast for 5 minutes, then serve.

NOTE If you can get hold of rainbow carrots, they really look great in this dish. Cauliflower also makes a great addition to the salad, just roast the florets along with the carrots in step 2.

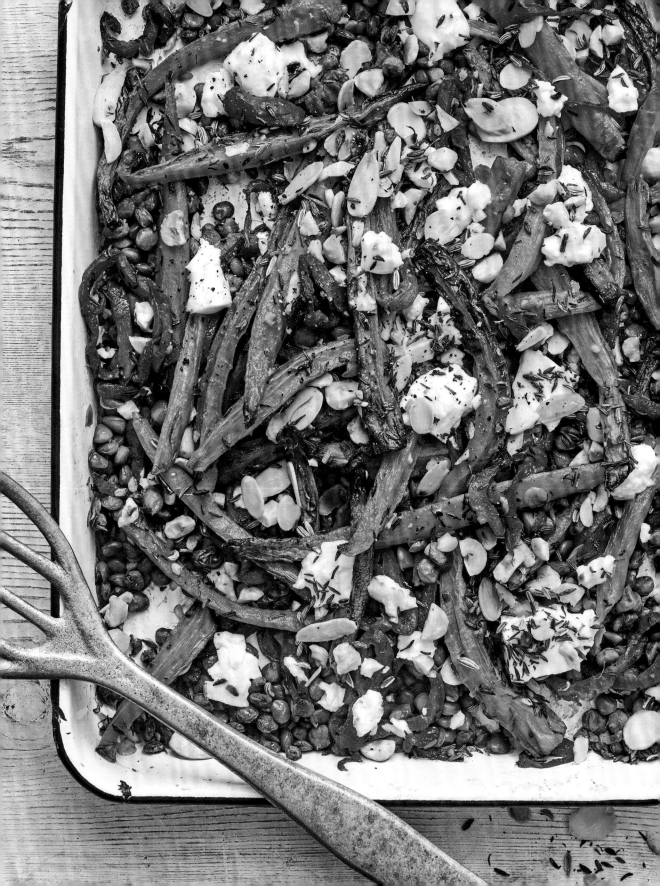

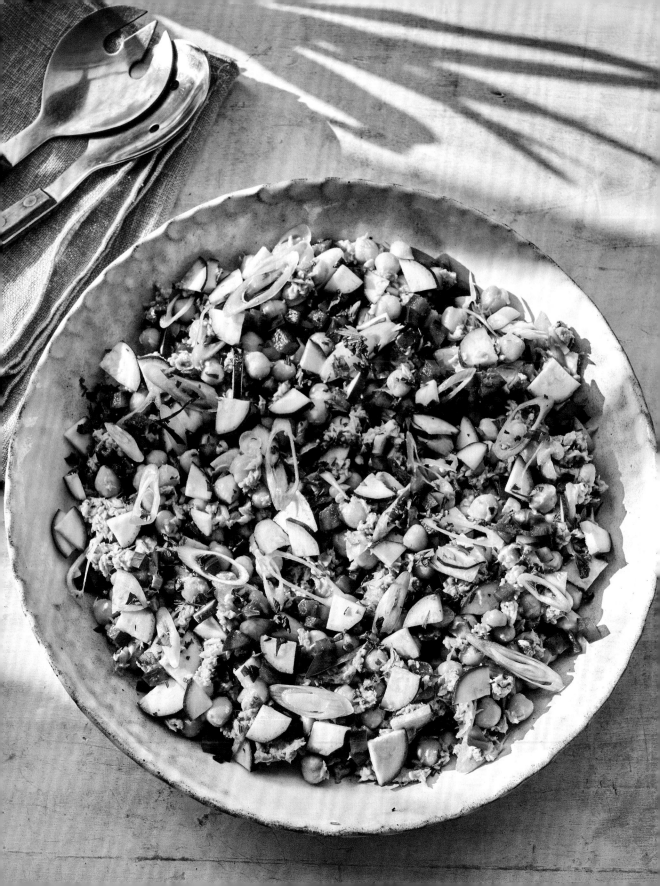

CHICKPEA & TUNA SALAD

I always keep tuna in the cupboard: it's a great salad ingredient and it has a long shelf life. This is quick to prepare, tasty and filling, using basic ingredients. It makes a great packed lunch, or a pitta bread or wrap filling. Canned tuna is ideal here, as it breaks down and coats the other ingredients. Fresh courgette and raw red pepper add nice crunch and splashes of colour, while a simple vinegar-mustard dressing brings it all together.

CALORIES PER SERVING: 125
PREP TIME: 10 MINUTES
COOK TIME: NONE

145g (5¼oz) can of tuna chunks
   in spring water, drained
1 tablespoon cider vinegar
1 teaspoon Dijon mustard
1 garlic clove, crushed
400g (14oz) can of chickpeas,
   drained and rinsed
1 red pepper, deseeded and finely
   chopped
1 small courgette, finely chopped
3 spring onions, finely sliced
small handful of parsley leaves,
   finely chopped
salt and pepper

1. In a large bowl, use a fork to mash the tuna up with the vinegar, mustard, garlic and some salt and pepper.
2. Mix in the chickpeas to fully coat with the tuna and dressing.
3. Add the red pepper, courgette, spring onions and parsley and toss them in.

NOTE Any crunchy, fresh vegetables that need using up will work well in this: you could add green beans, sugarsnap peas, broccoli, crunchy Iceberg lettuce, radishes or cucumber. You can also stir in some pre-cooked grains, such as bulgur wheat or couscous, to bulk this up.

CORONATION CHICKEN

This is my own take on coronation chicken, containing some of the key flavours but with more fresh vegetables added for crunch and flavour. (I could never stand the 'squishy' consistency of a lot of the coronation chicken I have been served in the past!) The slight cheat in this is using bought, pre-cooked chicken, but of course it would be an ideal recipe for using up roast chicken leftovers, too. I serve this with baked potatoes and salad, or just with pitta bread or crispbreads and salad. It's also great with the pre-cooked bags of mixed grains you can pick up at the supermarket.

CALORIES PER SERVING: 208
PREP TIME: 5 MINUTES
COOK TIME: NONE

350g (12oz) pre-cooked chicken
    breasts, skinned and finely
    chopped
1 red pepper, deseeded and finely
    chopped
2 spring onions, finely sliced
2 tablespoons light mayonnaise
6 tablespoons fat-free Greek
    yogurt
2 tablespoons mango chutney
2 teaspoons mild curry powder
1 teaspoon sweet or smoked
    paprika
salt and pepper

1. Simply mix all the ingredients together thoroughly, season with salt and pepper and serve.

NOTE This is a great recipe to use up some of those turkey leftovers at Christmas. You could also substitute the chicken for cooked prawns.

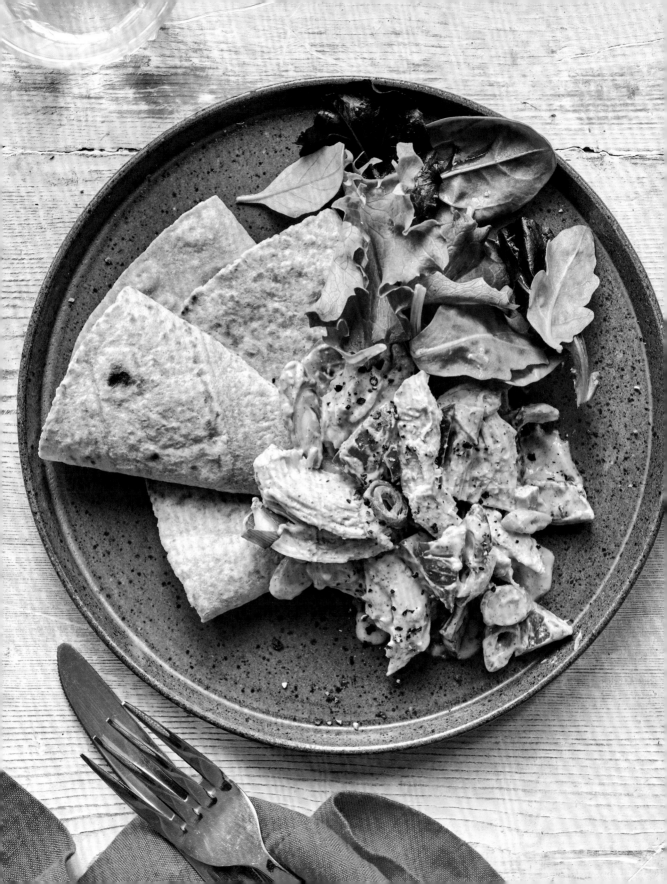

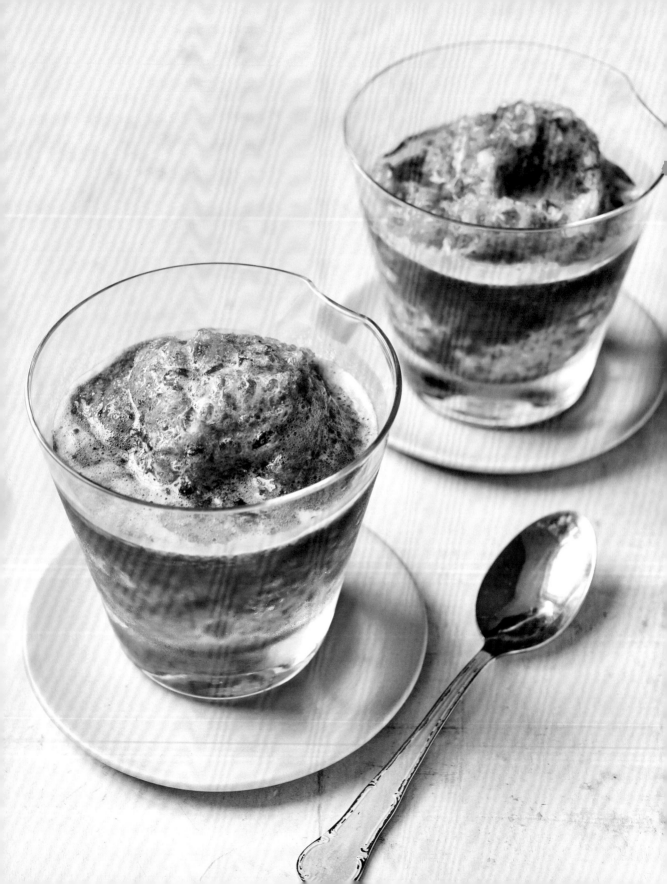

WHIPPED RASPBERRY WATER ICE

This refreshing dessert resembles a sorbet, but it's much lower in sugar and makes a great post-dinner sweet treat, or a cooling delight on a hot day.

CALORIES PER SERVING: 59
PREP TIME: 5 MINUTES, PLUS COOLING AND FREEZING TIME
COOK TIME: 10 MINUTES

60g (2¼oz) caster sugar
125ml (4fl oz) water
350g (12oz) frozen raspberries
2 egg whites

1. In a small saucepan, bring the sugar and measured water to the boil, then reduce the heat and allow to simmer for 3–5 minutes to fully dissolve the sugar.

2. Pour out of the pan into a small heatproof bowl and leave to cool fully: a little patience is required here! (You can speed up this process by placing the bowl of sugar syrup into a larger bowl of iced water.)

3. When the sugar syrup is cold, pour it into a food processor, add the frozen raspberries, and blend for about 1 minute until fully puréed (scrape down the sides halfway through blending to push down any bits that have stuck). Pour the egg whites into the food processor and whizz the mixture for about 1 minute: it will froth and whip up and just about double in size.

4. You can either serve as a soft-serve immediately, or pour the mixture into a 1-litre (1¾-pint) freezer-friendly container and freeze for 1-2 hours, depending on your desired consistency.

5. If freezing, remove from the freezer 10–20 minutes before serving to allow it to soften enough to scoop, or use a fork to rake it up granita-style.

NOTE Try a version of this with 350g (12oz) frozen mango and 1 passion fruit for an incredibly refreshing and tropical-tasting dessert.

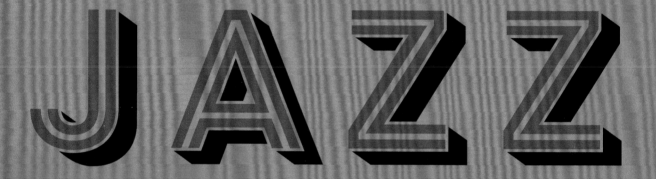

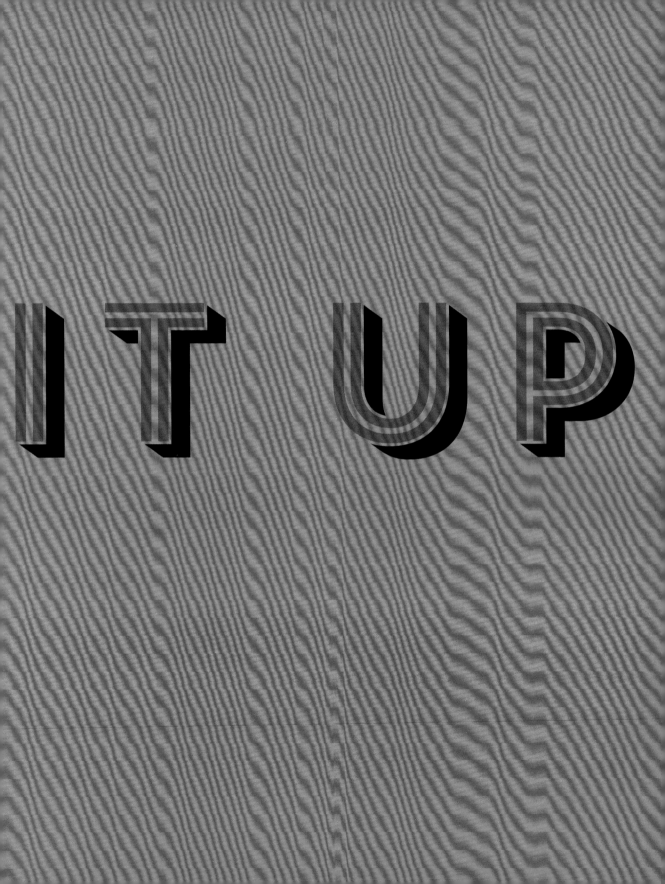

CHAPTER 7

WHOLEMEAL PITTA BREAD

So this one takes a *little* bit of a time investment, but it is worth it!
It is so useful and goes with pretty much any of the meals in this book.
Of course you can easily buy pitta bread, but this is on a whole different
level – so much nicer, plus you know exactly what went into them. Once
I have made a batch of these, any that are not eaten straight away are
frozen until I need them. The brilliant thing about frozen pitta bread is
that you can just pop it in the toaster to defrost, warm it up and add
a touch of crispness, then serve it straight away with soups, stews,
salads... These are also great to have in the freezer for those moments
when you discover the bread is mouldy; I often end up popping them
in the toaster to make up the kids' lunchboxes in the morning.

CALORIES PER PITTA: 110
PREP TIME: 15 MINUTES,
PLUS PROVING TIME
(1–2 HOURS)
COOK TIME: 5 MINUTES

175g (6oz) strong wholemeal
   bread flour, plus extra for
   dusting
75g (2¾oz) strong white bread
   flour
½ teaspoon fine sea salt
7g (2 teaspoons) fast-action
   dried yeast
140ml (4½fl oz) water, at room
   temperature

1. In a large bowl, mix up both flours, then add the salt,
   yeast and measured water. Use a knife to combine the
   ingredients, bringing them together to form a dough,
   then take over with your hands once the dough has
   started to come together and form it into a ball.

2. Transfer the dough to a work surface sprinkled with flour
   and knead it for 5 minutes (see box on page 205). It should
   feel almost silky to touch. Pop it back into the bowl, cover
   with a clean tea towel and leave (preferably in a warm
   place) to double in size (this should take approximately
   1–2 hours).

3. Preheat the oven to 240°C/220°C fan (475°F), Gas Mark 9.
   Remove the dough from the bowl and divide it into 8 pieces.
   Roll each piece into a ball, then sprinkle a work surface
   with flour once more and use a rolling pin to shape them
   into pitta breads (small ovals).

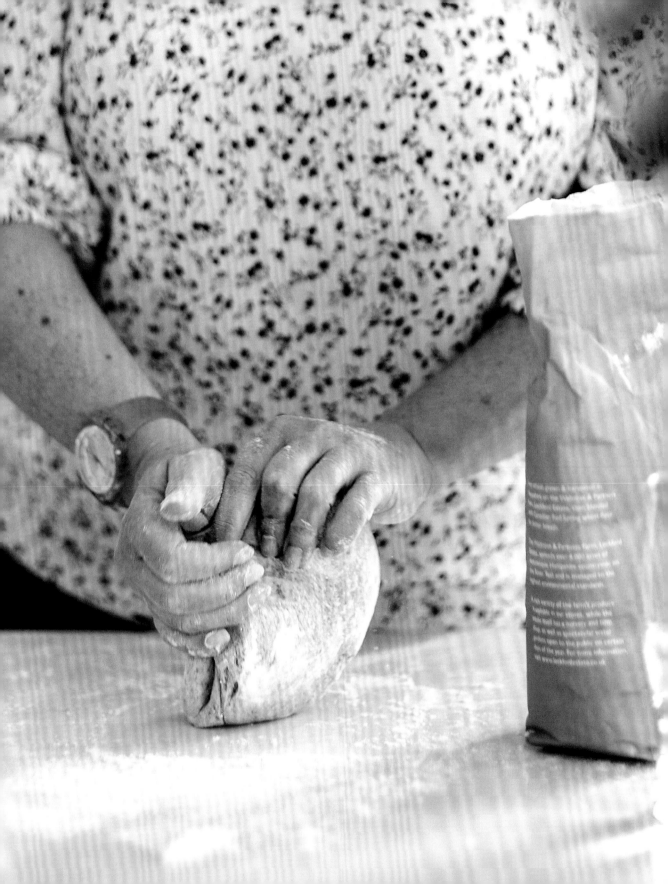

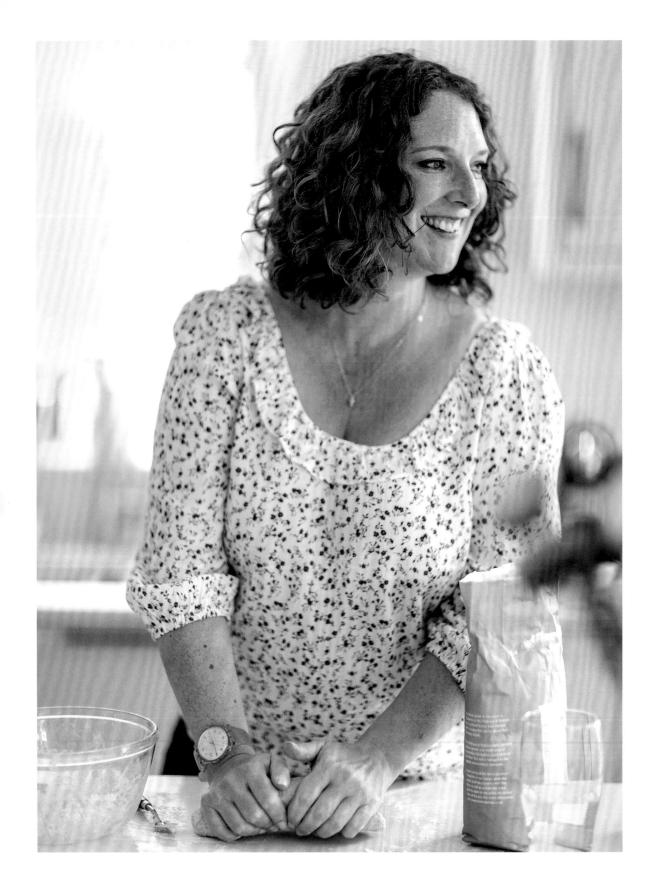

4. Space the breads out on a large baking tray and bake for 5 minutes. When you remove them from the oven they should be starting to go lightly golden brown and will be puffed up. If there is no golden colour, pop them back in for another minute or two, but be very careful not to burn them as they can turn very quickly!

5. If you aren't serving them immediately, wrap them in a clean tea towel until you need them, so they stay soft. You can warm them up again with a quick stint in the toaster if you need to.

HOW TO KNEAD
Start with a ball of dough and a lightly floured work surface. Use the palms of both hands to press the dough ball down and outward, stretching it out using the heels of your hands. Fold the dough in half back toward you and press down, then repeat the pushing down and out action. Keep on with this action, occasionally turning the dough 45 degrees. If the dough starts to feel a little bit sticky, sprinkle on a little extra flour. It will feel smooth and silky when it has been kneaded enough. With most doughs you will need to knead for at least 10 minutes, but with this one you can get away with five!

RED ONION CHUTNEY

A super-quick and easy, low-sugar chutney recipe which is great with cold cuts, cheeses, crackers, salads or curries. One of my favourite ways to use it is to spread it on seeded toast, cover with grated cheese and grill: the best-ever cheese on toast!

CALORIES PER SERVING: 68
PREP TIME: 10 MINUTES
COOK TIME: 40 MINUTES

1 teaspoon olive oil
6 red onions, finely chopped
400ml (14fl oz) apple juice
2 tablespoons light soft brown
 sugar
6 tablespoons balsamic vinegar
1 teaspoon salt

1. Heat the oil in a medium saucepan and fry the onions gently for 15 minutes, until soft.
2. Add the apple juice, sugar, balsamic vinegar and salt and simmer over a low heat for 30 minutes, stirring occasionally. The liquid should reduce and the chutney will thicken.
3. Transfer to a sterilized jar (see below) and store in the refrigerator for up to 1 month.

NOTE You can add a finely chopped red chilli to this for a bit of spice, in step 2.

TO STERILIZE JARS

Preheat the oven to 180°C/160°C fan (350°F), Gas Mark 4. Wash the jar in hot, soapy water, then rinse. Place upright on a baking tray, including the lid if separate (if you are using a jar with a rubber seal, remove this before putting the jar in the oven and boil it separately in a saucepan for 10 minutes to sterilize). Put the jars into the oven for 15 minutes, then allow to cool slightly before filling.

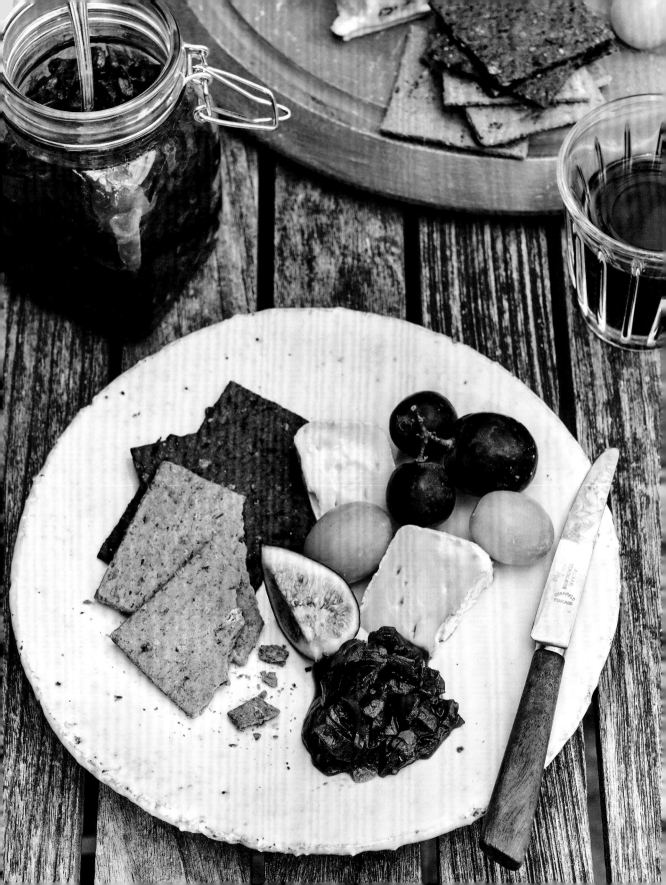

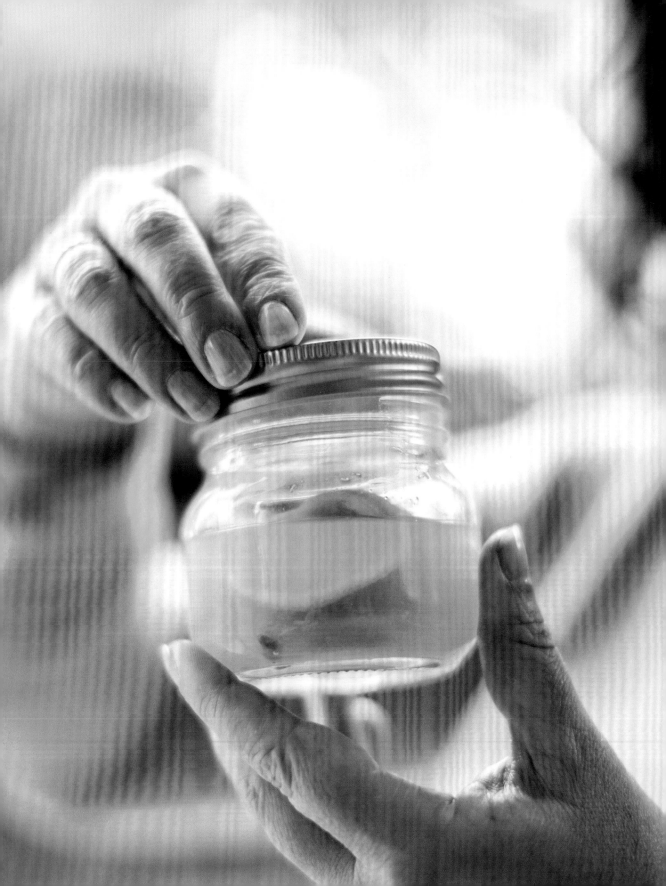

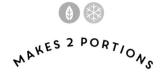

SPEEDY PRESERVED LEMONS

A brilliantly simple condiment which will quickly add bags of flavour to many different dishes. Found in many North African and Middle Eastern recipes, traditionally preserved lemons require weeks of patience before they are ready. I make a complete cheat's version, as I am rarely organized enough to preserve them the 'proper' way. This method will generate the amazing preserved lemon flavour in just 10 minutes. The downside is that they don't have the long shelf-life of traditional preserved lemons, but I just make one jar at a time and use it up within a week (if I haven't, I finely chop what's left and freeze it). Add them, finely chopped, to soups and stews, sprinkle over grilled meat or fish, pasta or salad, whizz into hummus or aioli, or stir into grains such as bulgur wheat or quinoa to add intense pops of zesty, savoury, lemony flavour.

CALORIES PER PORTION: 36
PREP TIME: 5 MINUTES, PLUS COOLING TIME
COOK TIME: 15 MINUTES

1 large, unwaxed lemon, washed, cut into 1cm (½ inch) slices, knobbly ends discarded
juice of 3 lemons
1 tablespoon coarse sea salt

1. In a small saucepan (with a lid), combine the lemon slices, lemon juice and salt, place over a high heat and gently stir to dissolve the salt (this will take about 1 minute).

2. Cover the pan with the lid, reduce the heat to low and gently simmer for 10 minutes. The peel on the lemon slices should become slightly translucent and feel tender when you poke it with a sharp knife. Give them a couple more minutes of simmering if they are still a bit tough.

3. Transfer to a sterilized jar (see page 206) and allow to cool slightly before screwing on the lid.

4. Keep in the refrigerator for up to 1 week. Any leftovers can be finely chopped, transferred to a small, airtight freezerproof container and frozen until needed.

QUICK PURPLE PICKLE

I make this regularly for adding some quick punchy flavour to lunches and dinners. It goes really well with pitta bread with grilled meat, fried halloumi, my Fakeaway Doner Kebab (see page 169), or it's great as a barbecue accompaniment, too. It's sharp and tangy with a cool mint flavour cutting through it.

CALORIES PER SERVING: 29
PREP TIME: 5 MINUTES
COOK TIME: NONE

1 large red onion, very finely
   sliced
small handful of mint leaves,
   finely chopped
1 red chilli, deseeded and finely
   chopped
2 tablespoons red wine vinegar
large pinch of salt

1. Pop everything into a small bowl and mix well. Keep for up to 2 weeks in the refrigerator

NOTE To bulk this out you can also add finely sliced red cabbage. Leave out the chilli if you don't want it spicy.

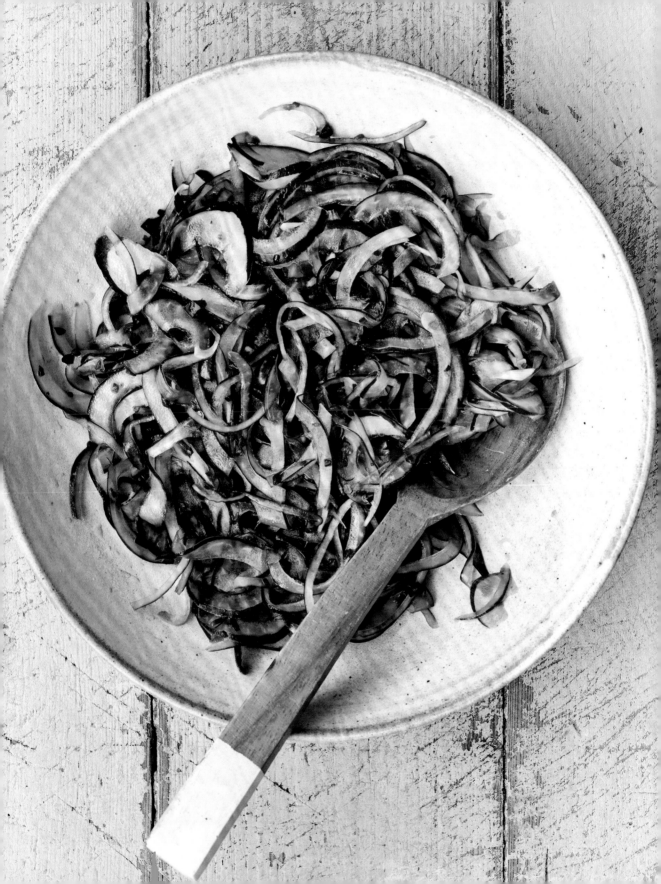

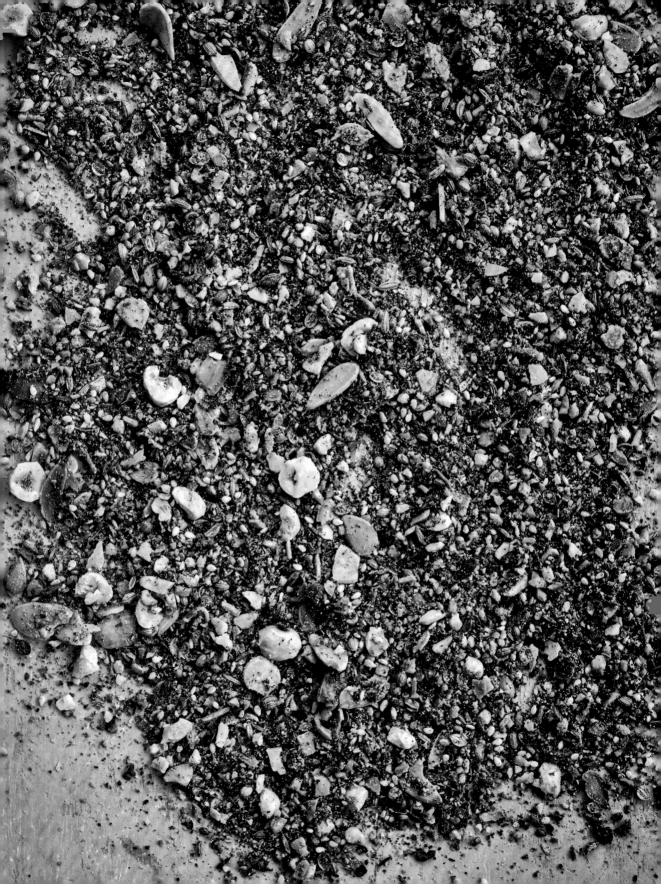

DUKKAH BLEND

Dukkah is a blend of nuts, seeds and spices, which originated in Egypt and has really grown in popularity in so many other countries over the past few years. You can pick up dukkah blends in many supermarkets now, but homemade dukkah tastes even better, and you can also tailor it to use nuts that you have in, or to your favourite flavours. I have used almonds and hazelnuts in my version but you could also try it with peanuts, pistachios, cashews or walnuts. Lightly toasting all the ingredients before blending adds so much flavour.

CALORIES PER TABLESPOON: 53
PREP TIME: 5 MINUTES
COOK TIME: 3 MINUTES

50g (1¾oz) blanched almonds
50g (1¾oz) blanched hazelnuts
2 tablespoons sesame seeds
1 tablespoon coriander seeds
1 tablespoon cumin seeds
½ tablespoon fennel seeds
1 teaspoon coarse sea salt

1. In a dry frying pan, toast the almonds and hazelnuts over a high heat for 2 minutes, shuffling them around in the pan to toast them all over.
2. Add the sesame, coriander, cumin and fennel seeds and fry for 1 more minute. Keep the heat high and use a wooden spoon or spatula to keep them moving in the pan for an even toast. Be on your guard, as sesame seeds can start to pop as they get hot!
3. Pour the mix into a mini chopper, add the salt and pulse-blend into a rough mix. Do this in short, sharp blasts so you don't accidentally purée everything: you want a rough texture.
4. Allow to cool, then transfer into a jar or airtight container. It will keep for up to 1 month.

HOW TO USE DUKKAH
A traditional Egyptian use is as a dip for flatbreads with olive oil, but it can liven up so many dishes.
- Sprinkle over hummus and dips.
- Add to salads or soups for extra texture and flavour.
- Scatter on cooked vegetables to liven them up.
- Use on grilled meat, fish, halloumi or tofu.
- Sprinkle over fried, poached or scrambled eggs.
- Use in my Roast Carrot & Lentil Salad with Feta & Dukkah (see page 192)

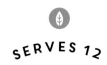

KETCHUP WITH A KICK

**Homemade ketchup is really easy to make and it's a great way
to have a healthier, lower-sugar alternative to the popular classic.
I make up a batch of this and keep in a sterilized (see page 206),
airtight 500ml (18fl oz) jar for up to 6 weeks in the refrigerator.
It's great for barbecues, bacon sarnies, serving up with sausages
and mash and even as a quick pizza sauce!**

CALORIES PER SERVING: 33
PREP TIME: 5 MINUTES, PLUS
COOLING TIME
COOK TIME: 25 MINUTES

2 × 400g (14oz) cans of chopped
   tomatoes
2 tablespoons red wine vinegar
3 tablespoons tomato purée
1 tablespoon Worcestershire
   sauce
1 tablespoon light brown sugar
1 teaspoon onion granules
1 teaspoon garlic granules
1 teaspoon salt
1 teaspoon chilli powder
¼ teaspoon mustard powder
¼ teaspoon allspice
¼ teaspoon pepper

1. Place all the ingredients into a medium-sized saucepan,
    bring up to a fast simmer and simmer for 25 minutes,
    stirring every now and again.
2. Use a hand blender or food processor to whizz into a
    smooth sauce. Transfer to a 500ml (18fl oz) sterilized
    airtight jar, allow to cool and keep in the refrigerator
    until needed for up to 6 weeks.

NOTE To make this without the kick, simply omit the chilli
powder when making the sauce.

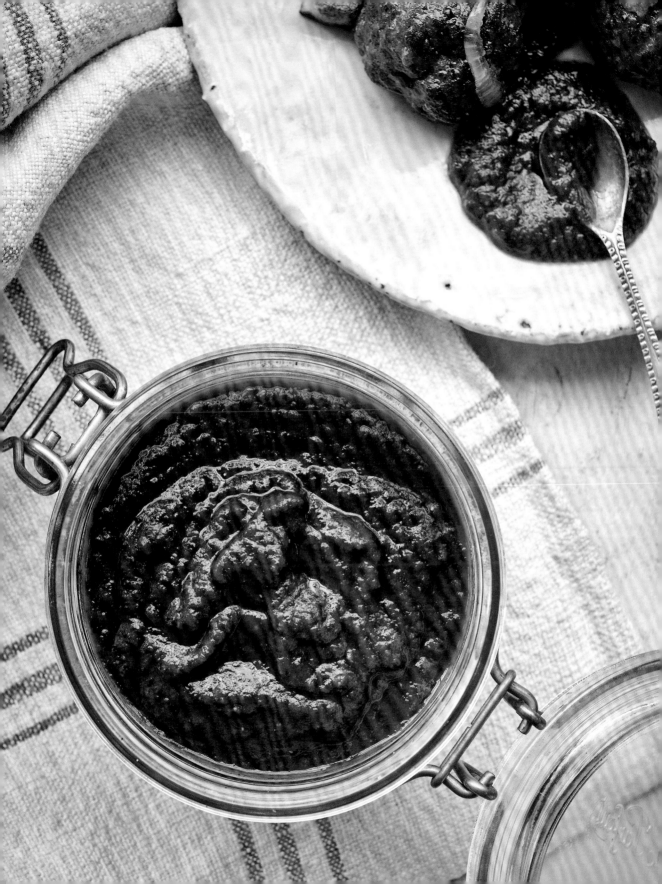

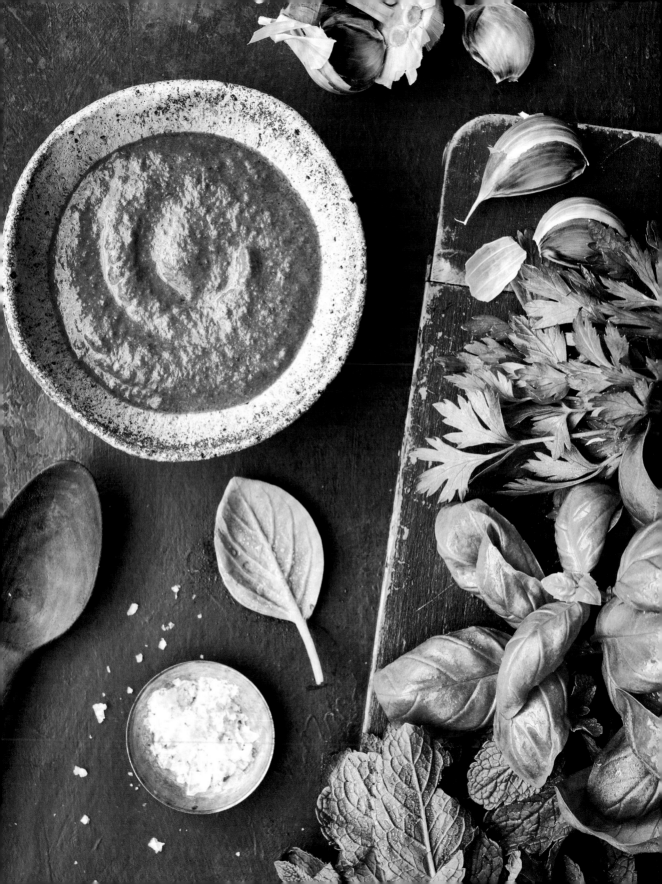

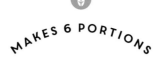

VEGGIE SALSA VERDE

I can remember really clearly the first time I tried salsa verde: my dad made it and served it with a really simple fried skate and I was blown away by how amazing it tasted! Traditional Italian salsa verde contains anchovies (and is utterly delicious), but I wanted to make a vegetarian version because you can still get such incredible flavour from it and it can be really versatile for jazzing up both veggie and meat dishes. I serve this with grilled meat or vegetables, over salads, with fried eggs, pasta, even spread in a sandwich or drizzled over a pizza. It is also a great way to use up leftover herbs before they spoil. You will need a mini chopper to make this – a really useful and fairly low-cost bit of kitchen equipment – though some hand blenders have an attachment for a mini chopper function.

CALORIES PER SERVING: 16
PREP TIME: 5 MINUTES
COOK TIME: NONE

1 large garlic clove, roughly
   chopped
2 large handfuls of flat leaf
   parsley leaves
large handful of basil leaves
small handful of mint leaves
1 tablespoon capers
1 teaspoon Dijon mustard
2 tablespoons red wine vinegar
1 teaspoon olive oil
1 ice cube
salt and pepper

1. Put all the ingredients in a mini chopper and purée until smooth and spoonable. The reason for the ice is to keep all the ingredients cold, which retains a vivid green colour in the salsa.

NOTE There are no weights included here for the herbs because it isn't a precise science: typically parsley is the herb used in the greatest quantities, but it is really something you can play around with to find your perfect balance. You might wish to use up a big amount of a specific herb, or tailor it to something that you are cooking. Just taste as you go and experiment until it is perfect for you.

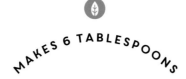

CRUNCHY SEED SPRINKLE

(SAVOURY OR SWEET)

This is magic, one of my secret weapons for jazzing up lots of sweet and savoury dishes. The salty soy version is perfect over rice and grains, curries, salads, grilled vegetables or meat, just to add a new texture and another layer of flavour. The sweet maple sprinkle is lovely on porridge, scattered over yogurt and fruit, or on rice pudding. Once I have made these, I keep them for up to 1 month in an airtight jar or pot so they are on hand whenever I need them.

CALORIES PER SERVING:
86 (SOY)/92 (MAPLE SYRUP)
PREP TIME: 5 MINUTES
COOK TIME: 4 MINUTES

2 tablespoons pumpkin seeds
2 tablespoon golden linseeds
2 tablespoons sunflower seeds
2 tablespoons chia seeds
1 tablespoon dark soy sauce
    (savoury) OR 1 tablespoon
    pure maple syrup (sweet)

1. In a medium-sized frying pan, toast the seeds over a high heat for 2 minutes, shuffling them around with a wooden spoon every now and again to prevent burning.

2. After 2 minutes, you'll be able to smell that lovely toastiness. Take the pan off the heat and immediately add the soy sauce or maple syrup, quickly stirring it through all the seeds. Keep mixing while the liquid evaporates and the seeds pick up the flavour.

3. Leave to cool completely, then stir again to break down any clumps that have formed. Transfer into an airtight container to store for up to 1 month.

NOTE Beware of spitting: the linseeds can burst and spit while they are toasting, so be on your guard!

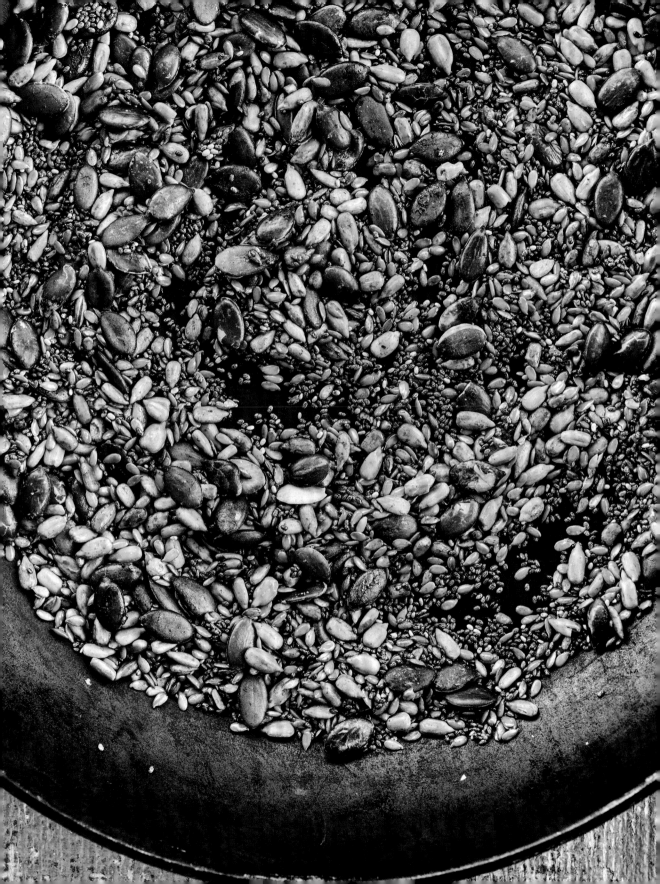

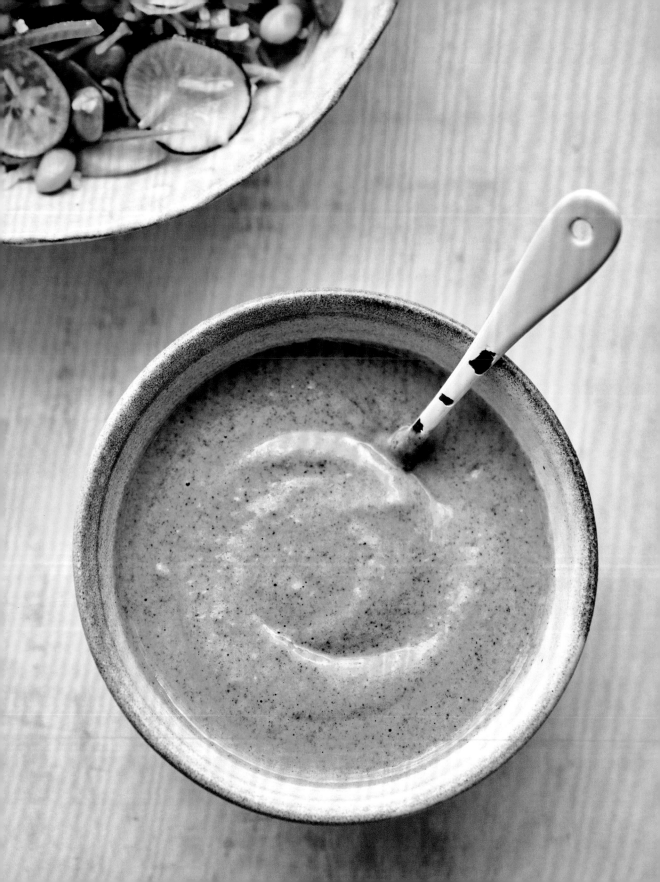

YUM-YUM SAUCE

A Japanese/American-inspired pink sauce, almost like a prawn cocktail sauce in appearance. The mix of flavours means it is very versatile, and although I tend to pair it with Crunchy Japanese-Style Rice Salad with Yum-Yum Sauce (see page 187), you can drizzle it over noodles, use it as a dipping sauce for vegetables or French fries, or serve it as a sauce for grilled meat or seafood. This would normally be made with mayonnaise, but I have used an aioli-style base to keep it light on calories while retaining a creamy consistency.

CALORIES PER SERVING: 76
PREP TIME: 5 MINUTES
COOK TIME: NONE

1 medium egg
150g (5½oz) fat-free Greek yogurt
1 tablespoon tomato purée
1 tablespoon white rice vinegar
1 tablespoon honey
½ teaspoon sweet paprika
½ teaspoon garlic granules
½ teaspoon onion granules
½ teaspoon cayenne pepper
¼ teaspoon salt

1. In a medium-sized bowl, whisk the egg, then whisk in the yogurt.
2. Add all the remaining ingredients and whisk everything together until you have a smooth sauce.
3. Serve immediately, or keep in the refrigerator until you are ready to use it (for up to 5 days).

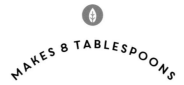

TANDOORI-STYLE SPICE BLEND

I used to turn to a pre-made Tandoori spice blend, because it's such an easy way to get great flavour into meat and fish. By having your own mix made up, you can use it as a seasoning, or mix it with yogurt to marinate chicken or fish.

CALORIES PER TABLESPOON: 18
PREP TIME: 5 MINUTES
COOK TIME: NONE

1 tablespoon ground ginger
1 tablespoon ground cumin
1 tablespoon ground coriander
1 tablespoon sweet paprika
2 teaspoons ground turmeric

2 teaspoons fine sea salt
2 teaspoons garlic granules
2 teaspoons onion granules
1 teaspoon cayenne pepper

1. Combine all the ingredients together and store in a jam jar or other airtight container. This will keep for up to 6 months.

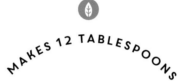

GREEK-STYLE SEASONING

This is a winner to have made up ready because it is so versatile! Use it for my Lemon & Herb Roast Chicken Dinner (see page 116), or simply as a seasoning for any meat, fish or vegetables that need a bit of a Mediterranean flavour injection.

CALORIES PER TABLESPOON: 23
PREP TIME: 5 MINUTES
COOK TIME: NONE

3 tablespoons dried oregano
2 tablespoons onion granules
2 tablespoons garlic granules
1 tablespoon dried basil
1 tablespoon dried dill

1 tablespoon dried rosemary
½ tablespoon dried thyme
½ tablespoon fine sea salt
½ tablespoon pepper

1. Combine all the ingredients together and store in a jam jar or other airtight container. This will keep for up to 6 months.

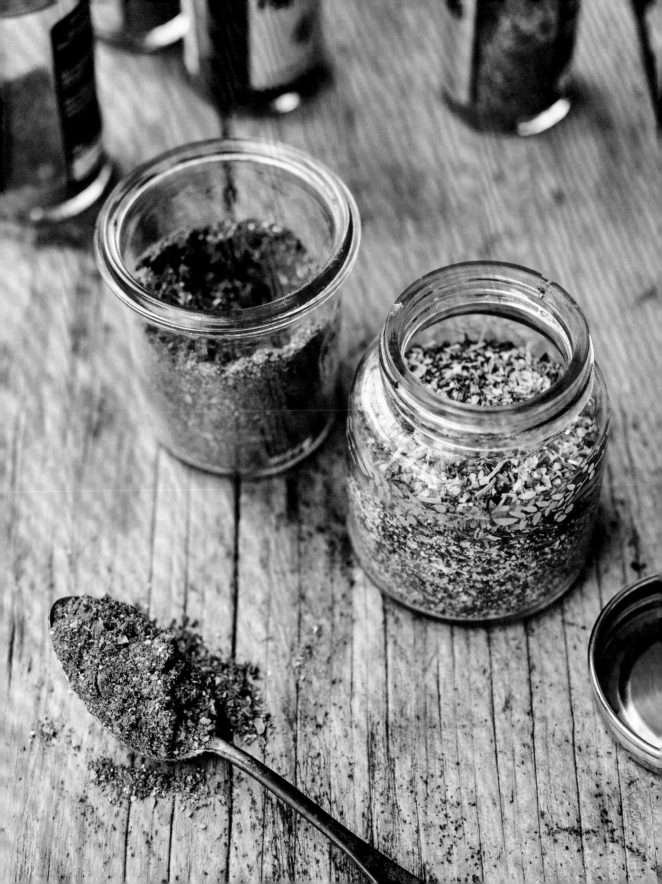

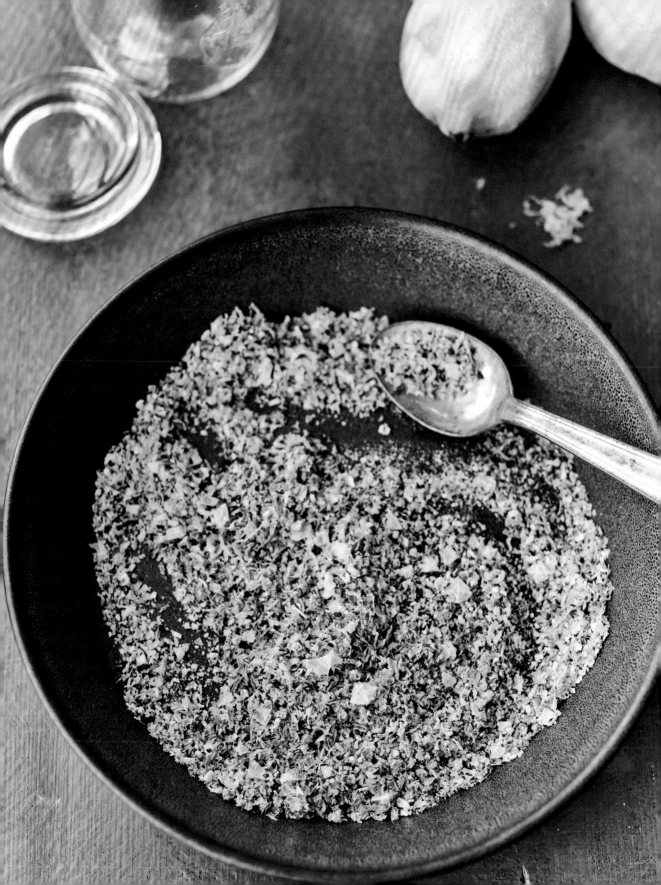

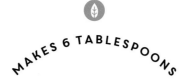

LEMON PEPPER

A handy little mix to have around. Not only is it great in meals such as Chicken Lemon Pepperpot (see page 31), but it can be used as a stand-alone seasoning for chicken and fish, or beef, potato wedges, roast cauliflower, pasta salad or green vegetables, adding tangy flavour and deep, satisfying warmth.

CALORIES PER TABLESPOON: 23
PREP TIME: 5 MINUTES
COOK TIME: 40 MINUTES

3 unwaxed lemons
2 tablespoons pepper
1 tablespoon salt
1 tablespoon onion granules
1 tablespoon garlic granules

1. Preheat the oven to 120°C/100°C fan (250°F), Gas Mark ½.
2. Line a baking tray with baking parchment and finely grate the zest of all 3 lemons directly on to this until you have removed all the zest.
3. Place on the middle shelf of the oven for 40 minutes (check on it after 30 minutes to make sure it isn't browning). The zest should be crisp to the touch but not burned or browned. Remove from the oven and tip the zest into a small bowl.
4. Add the remaining ingredients and mix thoroughly.
5. Store in a jam jar or other airtight container for up to 1 year.

> **CHEAT'S LEMON PEPPER**
> Lemon pepper is not commonly available to buy, so if you don't have time to make your own, simply replace it with 1 tablespoon freshly ground black pepper, 1 teaspoon salt and the finely grated zest of 1 unwaxed lemon.
>
> **GREATER GRATING**
> I thoroughly recommend investing in a Microplane for zesting fruit and grating Parmesan cheese. It makes it so quick to shave off that lovely top layer of zest, as well as making light work of a pile of snowy grated Parmesan.

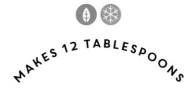

MASALA CURRY PASTE

Having a curry paste ready prepared is a great way to be able to knock up a curry in a hurry! Use this paste for tangy Lemon Chicken with Masala Chickpeas (see page 76). This recipe can easily be scaled up if you wish. I keep it in an airtight jar in the refrigerator for up to 5 days and, if I haven't used it by then, I transfer it into a small plastic container and freeze until I need it.

CALORIES PER SERVING: 25
PREP TIME: 5 MINUTES
COOK TIME: NONE

2 onions, quartered
8 garlic cloves, roughly chopped
65g (2¼oz) fresh root ginger, peeled and roughly chopped
2 green chillies, stalks discarded, roughly chopped
2 tablespoons ground cumin
1 tablespoon ground coriander
2 teaspoons chilli powder
2 teaspoons ground turmeric
1 teaspoon ground cinnamon
1 teaspoon pepper
1 teaspoon salt
2 tablespoons red wine vinegar
juice of 1 lemon

1. Simply put all the ingredients in a mini chopper or small food processor and blend into a smooth paste. Transfer into an airtight container and store in the refrigerator for up to 5 days, or freeze until needed.

NOTE This paste will work well with meat, fish, vegetables or pulses for a great curry every time. Simply gently fry the paste for a couple of minutes, then add your ingredients of choice with some chicken or vegetable stock. If you want to make it a creamy curry, add a 400ml (14fl oz) can of light coconut milk, or just some fat-free yogurt.

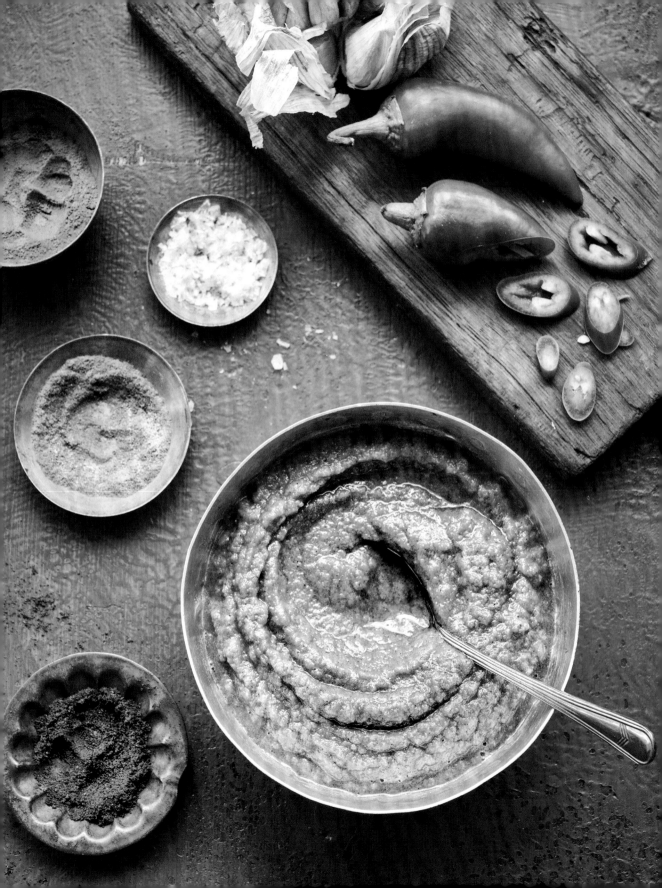

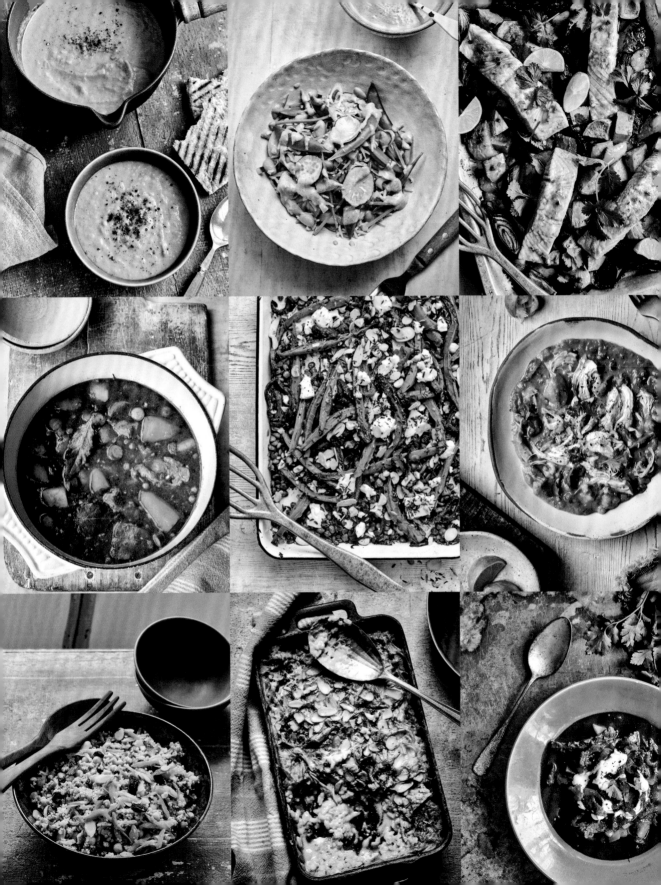

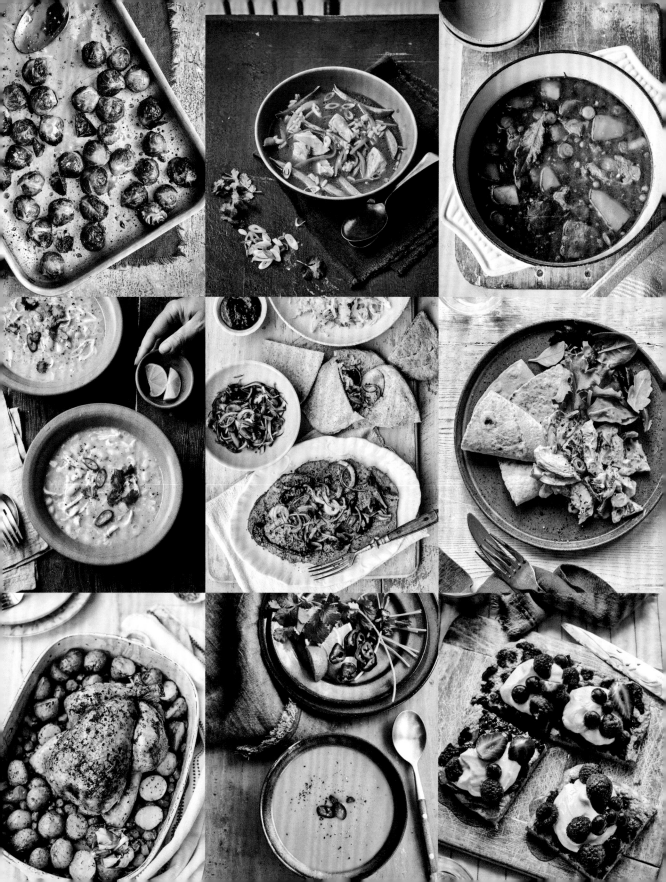

GLOSSARY

UK	US
aubergine	eggplant
baking parchment	parchment paper
butter beans	lima beans
caster sugar	superfine sugar
chilli flakes	red pepper flakes
coriander	cilantro
cornflour	cornstarch
courgette	zucchini
garlic and herb roulé soft cheese	full-fat soft cheese with garlic and herbs
green beans	string beans
green pepper/red pepper/ yellow pepper	bell peppers
grill	broil
haricot beans	navy beans
muslin	cheesecloth
rocket	arugula
samphire	sea asparagus/beach asparagus
semi-skimmed milk	1.5–1.8 per cent fat milk
spring onions	scallions
tomato passata	smooth tomato sauce
tomato purée	tomato paste
wholemeal	wholegrain

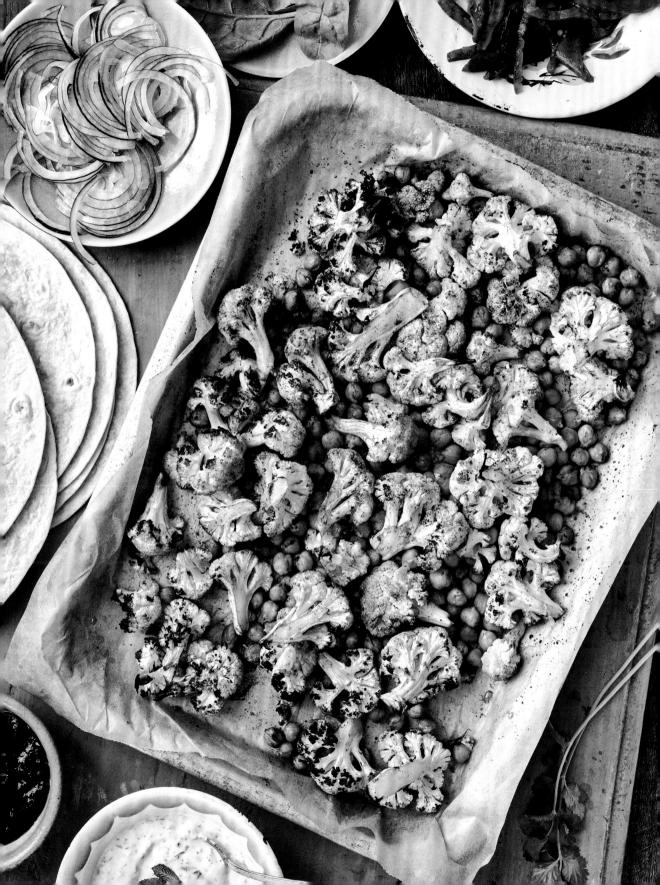

INDEX

RECIPE LIST

AUTHOR'S ACKNOWLEDGEMENTS

It's so hard to know where to start when so many hard-working people have been involved in bringing this book together, but I will start close to home. Thank you to my family, who mean absolutely everything to me. My husband Darren, for always encouraging me to step out of my comfort zone and without whom I would never have had the confidence to start a blog (for which he acts as web developer, technical support, designer, cameraman and chief taste-tester!) I couldn't have done this without you.

Thank you to my daughters, Miette and Marlie, you are the reason that I always have my sights set high and want to be a success. My sweet, kind, caring, funny girls; thank you for being so understanding when I am constantly stressed during recipe-testing time, and when it means I miss out on days at the beach and holiday fun. I am so very proud of you both.

Thank you to my Mum and Dad for everything you have done for me, including helping us out in the tough times, I am very grateful for you both.

With an intense period of recipe-testing comes a need for willing food-testers, and thanks to my lovely, supportive neighbours/friends for willingly taking on multiple containers of food, and for always asking how the book's going, and showing so much support.

Thank you to my agent, Heather Holden-Brown, for sharing your experience and wisdom with me.

The strange times of 2020 and 2021 have meant that I still haven't met most of the brilliant team who are responsible for making this book come to life, but I appreciate what a huge, complicated and pressured undertaking it is, and I have been lucky enough to spend time with my Commissioning Editor, Natalie Bradley, who 'got' what The Slimming Foodie is from the very start, and has allowed me to stick my oar in a lot more than maybe some authors would! Thank you also to Art Director Yasia Williams for listening to me, and for bringing together everything on the art and design side of things, and to both of you for being great fun at the photoshoots.

Thanks to those of you at Octopus: Katherine Hockley, Hazel O'Brien, Karen Baker, Kevin Hawkins and to everyone who I haven't met but I know are integral cogs in this process. Thank you again to Lucy Bannell for copyediting my manuscript, to Senior Managing Editor Sybella Stephens for whipping everything into shape, and to Grade Design.

I was so thrilled to be able to reassemble the brilliant shoot team from book one. Thank you Chris Terry for the beautiful photographs, and for making the shoot such fun, as well as making sure that we are kept well fed with coffee, doughnuts and poke bowls! I was also so happy that Tamsin Weston was again Props Stylist – your impeccable taste shines throughout the book, and working with you is an absolute pleasure every time. Henrietta Clancy deserves special recognition for the food styling whilst heavily pregnant, which must have been utterly exhausting, but you still made it through an hugely impressive amount of dishes every day, and were fantastic company. I will never forget your grand entrance on day one with the Beef bourguignon! Thanks also to Sophie Denmead for being the Assistant Food Stylist for most of the shoot, and again for being so lovely to work with. Many thanks also to Octavia Squire for doing a brilliant job of styling week one food, and to Georgie Besterman for holding the fort during week two.

Last, but definitely not least, thank-you so much to all of you who follow me on social media, use the blog recipes and who bought the first book. Reading the lovely reviews of book 1, seeing all of the dishes being brought to life in your homes, and finding out which of the recipes were your favourites was a true highlight of 2021. Thank you for keeping everything positive on my social media channels, I feel very lucky to be part of such a supportive community.

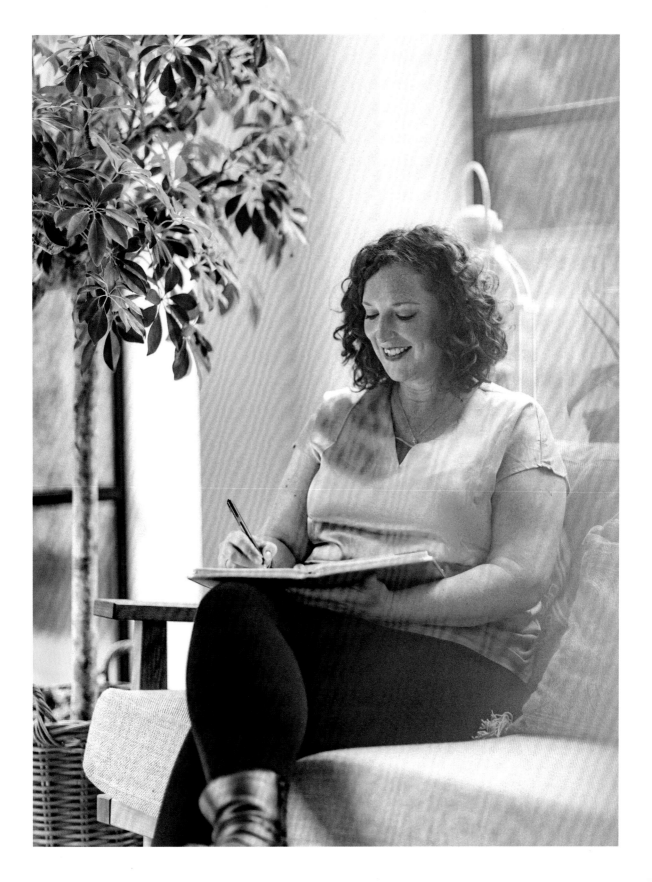

ABOUT THE AUTHOR

Pip Payne is behind the award-winning blog The Slimming Foodie, which she started in 2015 to share lighter takes on her favourite dishes. Keeping a love of food at the fore, Pip's approach is about bringing back convenient home cooking by making healthy recipes that are accessible to a new wave of home cooks.

Pip lives in Devon with her husband, two daughters and their dog.

www.theslimmingfoodie.com
@ @the_slimming_foodie

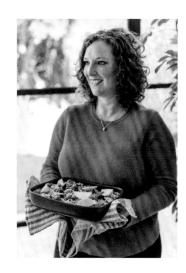

ALSO BY PIP PAYNE

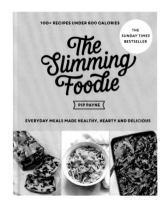

The Slimming Foodie